Skinny Bitch:
Bun in the Oven

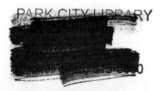

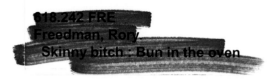
Skinny Bitch:
Bun in the Oven

*A Gutsy Guide to Becoming
One Hot and Healthy Mother!*

By Rory Freedman and Kim Barnouin

RUNNING PRESS
PHILADELPHIA · LONDON

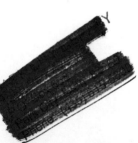

9   8   7   6   5   4   3   2   1
Digit on the right indicates the number of this printing

Library of Congress Control Number: 2008930504

ISBN 978-0-7624-3105-2

Cover design and interior design by Amanda Richmond
Edited by Jennifer Kasius
Typography: Bodoni, Dutch, and Helvetica Neue.

Note: This book is intended only as an informative guide for those wishing to know more
about health issues. In no way is this book intended to replace, countermand, or conflict
with the advice given to you by your own physician. The ultimate decision concerning care
should be made between you and your doctor. We strongly recommend you follow his or
her advice.

Running Press Book Publishers
2300 Chestnut Street
Philadelphia, PA 19103-4371

Visit us on the web!
www.runningpress.com

Contents

Acknowledgments

We're so fortunate and thankful to work with such talented, committed people: Talia Cohen, Laura Dail, Jennifer Kasius, Jon Anderson, Seta Zink, Craig Herman, Melissa Appleby, Peter Costanzo, Amanda Richmond, Margarete Gockel, Victoria Gilder, Isabelle Bleecker, David Steinberger, the entire sales team, and everyone else at Running Press and Perseus.

For your wisdom, input, and generosity, we cannot thank you enough: Dina Aronson, MS, RD, Dr. Jessica Schneider, Dr. Scott Cohen, Dr. Kimberly Klausner, Dr. Guy Efron, Dr. David Ghozland, Dianne Van Treeck, MS, RD, CDE, Patti Howard, Dr. Neal Barnard, Dr. Hope Ferdowsian, Dr. Michael Greger, Dr. Gary Fraser, Dr. Jennifer Prescott, Eric Prescott, Jerry Friedman, Ilana Sparrow, and Bruce Friedrich.

Special thanks and love to Chloé Jo Berman, James Costa, Karen Coyne, Jackie Poper, Gretchen Ryan, Lauren Silverman, Tracy Silverman, Tim VanOrden, Meri Freedman, Rick Freedman, Tim, Maya, and Lesley Bailey, Anna Werderitsch, L.Ac., John Newton, and Stephane and Jackson Barnouin.

*For mothers
(especially single mothers), who
are the unsung heroes of the world.*

---

*And for our own mothers,
with the deepest love and gratitude.*

Foreword

AS AN OB/GYN WITH A FULL OBSTETRICAL PRACTICE, I see many women with concerns about their diet during pregnancy. If you are looking to make small changes in your diet, this is a helpful, educational guide for making healthier choices. If you are looking to make more radical changes but not sure how or where to start, the varied and delicious menu plan can really help you jumpstart the process. Rory and Kim manage to be straightforward, entertaining, and very thought-provoking all at the same time.

Whether you are looking for a few tips or an overhaul in your eating plan, this book is an incredibly useful guide. Pregnancy is a special and unique time, and can be the perfect motivation for doing something to improve your health and how you feel. The best thing you can do for your baby is to take care of yourself, and it is never too late to do something about your own health and well-being.

Jessica Lynn Schneider, MD, FACOG
Obstetrics and Gynecology

AS A PEDIATRICIAN, I CAN HAPPILY SAY THAT *Skinny Bitch: Bun in the Oven* outlines a safe, healthy diet for pregnant women and their babies. Rory and Kim's brash language is down-to-earth and makes for an entertaining read. Their anecdotes and thorough research will force you to ask questions and examine your daily life.

In my practice, families commonly ask me about lifestyle choices. In pediatrics, parents are accustomed to hearing many different ways to do the same thing. For example, if you asked twenty people how to introduce solid foods to their infant, or train them to sleep through the night, or how to treat the common cold, you would likely receive twenty different responses. As a result, I teach "common sense pediatrics" or "common sense parenting." We may not always agree on what to do for our children, but we should agree that there is more than one right way. *Skinny Bitch: Bun in the Oven* presents one of these "right" ways—the advantages of a vegan lifestyle during pregnancy and beyond.

Scott W. Cohen, MD, FAAP
Pediatrics

Introduction

Congratulations. You're knocked up. Chances are, you've dreamt of being pregnant since you were a little girl. So take a moment to acknowledge that you are living a dream and be thankful. Okay, that's enough. You've got work to do. Being a good mother starts now. Unless you were raised by crackheads, you know that your diet is the most important factor in determining your baby's health. Indeed, it's an awesome responsibility, but don't let it overwhelm you. It's not rocket science. While there are a few specific things pregnant women do need to adhere to, overall, you just need to be healthy. Healthy mommy=healthy baby. So feel doubly blessed because your pregnancy will force you to finally prioritize your own well-being. Get psyched: you are about to embark on the most exciting journey of your lifetime—motherhood and optimal health!

BITCHCLAIMER

We didn't write this book to make friends. We wrote this book to help women eat right—ensuring successful pregnancies and healthy babies. So if you want to hear "everything in moderation," "an occasional glass of wine is fine," or any other candy-coated bullshit, pick another book. We will tell you the truth about food and how what you eat affects your pregnancy and baby.

Go make friends at your Lamaze classes. We're invested in making a difference in your life.

P.S. This isn't *What to Expect When You're Expecting*. We don't provide a blow-by-blow of what's happening each month, and we don't give you the lowdown on the best burp cloths. It's a how-to-eat guide, with a few extras here and there.

P.P.S. A healthy pregnancy diet isn't drastically different than a healthy regular diet. So if you read our first book, *Skinny Bitch*, don't be surprised (or pissed) to find much of the same information here.

P.P.P.S. We're not gynos, so be sure to talk to your doctor about any of our recommendations.

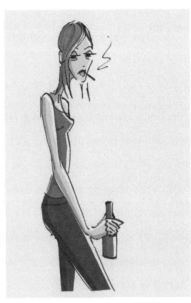

Chapter One

You're Knocked Up, Now Give It Up

Use your head. If you want a healthy baby, you have to be healthy. Which means you have to give up your gross vices. Not only is smoking N-A-S-T-Y, but it can cause premature birth, attention deficit disorder (ADD) during childhood, asthma, respiratory disease, and low birth weight. All the toxic components from smoking go directly into your baby's bloodstream, weakening the immune system. This also constricts the veins and arteries, which decreases the flow of oxygen, blood, and nutrients to your baby. Women who smoke are at least twenty times more likely to miscarry than nonsmokers.[1] Give it up. And steer clear of secondhand smoke, too.

Ditto for drinking. Just two drinks a day can significantly increase your risk of miscarriage.[2] Alcohol enters the fetal bloodstream in the same concentration it enters yours. But it takes the baby twice as long to eliminate the alcohol from his system. Drinking while pregnant can cause low birth weight, premature labor, mental deficiencies, physical deformities, and even neonatal death.[3] Alcohol can cause pre- and postnatal growth deficiencies, congenital heart defects, brain anomalies, and an atypical facial appearance.[4] Abnormalities can be seen in approximately one-third of infants born to heavy drinkers. And heavy drinking doesn't mean a bottle of Jack Daniels. It means only an average of one ounce or more of alcohol per day.[5] If you are craving wine, beer, or booze while pregnant, you're in trouble. To get help quitting drinking, call the Alcoholics Anonymous World Headquarters at 212-870-3400 to find an AA meeting near you or visit www.alcoholics-anonymous.org. (Don't be afraid. It'll make you a better mom and a happier person.) If you hit the bottle before you knew you were pregnant, don't beat yourself up. Just make healthy choices from here on out.

And stop injecting coffee into your veins! Caffeine is a diuretic (it makes you pee more), and it drains fluid and calcium from the body,[6] both of which are vital to mom and baby. It can also interfere with your body's ability to absorb iron, which is also detrimental.[7] Now, we know nothing incites rage like suggesting someone kick his or her coffee habit. Time and time again, we see how resistant people are to giving it up.

Make no mistake: coffee is a highly addictive drug for many people. And like all drugs, it comes with an ugly slew of side effects. Caffeine (whether found in coffee, tea, or soda) can cause headaches, digestive problems, irritation of the stomach and bladder, peptic ulcers, diarrhea, constipation, fatigue, anxiety, and depression. It affects every organ system, from the nervous system to the skin. Caffeine raises stress hormone levels, inhibits important enzyme systems that are responsible for cleaning the body, and sensitizes nerve reception sites.[8] It basically puts the body into a "fight or flight" mode every time you drink it, so imagine how it can affect your unborn baby: decreased birth weight, smaller head size, jitters, metabolic problems, and even mental retardation.[9] Add its potential to worsen mood swings and affect your sleep,[10] and it becomes really difficult to see the point. Not convinced? Even moderate consumption can affect fetal heart rate and movement patterns.[11] In infants, caffeine can cause rapid respiration, tremors, and the development of diabetes later in life. In countries with the highest rates of diabetes, the caffeine consumption is highest, too. It's suspected that the buildup of caffeine in the fetal pancreas can cause damage to insulin-producing cells.[12] Happy Birthday, junior! I got you some diabetes! Here's our last-ditch effort: If drinking more than two cups of coffee a day increases the likelihood of miscarriage,[13] why would you mess with one? IT'S JUST NOT WORTH IT. GET OVER YOUR ADDICTION. It'll be a tough week or two, and then you'll be free for life.

We are sympathetic if you're already hooked. Just do your best to immediately start weaning yourself off. Start by blending your regular coffee with decaf. If you make coffee at home, mix together three-quarters regular and one-quarter decaf coffee beans. If you get your java at a coffee shop, ask them to mix it for you. In three days, do half regular, half decaf. In another three days, do one-quarter regular and three-quarters decaf. Three days later, say goodbye to your regular and go full throttle on the decaf. But just for five days. Each day, try to leave a little bit more left in your cup so that by the end of the week, you can walk away from your decaf, too. You don't want to replace your regular coffee addiction with a decaf addiction.

Coffee beans, like other crops, are grown with chemical pesticides. And decaffeinating them doesn't get rid of the pesticides. In fact, sometimes, the decaffeination process can actually incorporate more chemicals! One compound, methylene chloride, is also used as an industrial solvent and paint stripper, and chronic exposure may cause birth defects.[14]

A better way to start the day is with a hot cup of lemon water. It's great for getting started on your water intake for the day, and there's the bonus of a little vitamin C from the fresh lemon juice. Or have a glass of juice, for crying out loud. That's the kind of morning buzz that won't come with any negative side effects.

Speaking of negative side effects: When your newborn arrives, will you put soda into a baby bottle and feed it to her? So why would you feed it to her in utero? Soda is garbage for both of your bodies; just say "no" to this liquid Lucifer. Pregnant women need an additional 200 to 300 calories a day in their second and third trimesters but these need to come from wholesome foods with nutritional value. Soda offers no value whatsoever. You might as well stick your head in the toilet bowl and drink from there. (Don't even get us started on caffeine-infused "energy" drinks. Those are the friggin' anti-Christ.) Soda is loaded with caffeine and has the equivalent of ten teaspoons of sugar![15] In addition, it can cause excessive abdominal fat, high blood pressure, reduction of good cholesterol, an increased risk of obesity, and can lead to heart disease and diabetes. By the way, this is regular *and* diet soda we're talking about here![16] So don't go patting yourself on the back if you drink diet soda. That stuff is even worse. It's not good for you (pregnant or not), and it's sure as hell not good for your baby. Artificial sweeteners like aspartame (Equal or NutraSweet) contain aspartic acid, phenylalanine, and methanol, all of which may cause abnormalities in the brains of developing fetuses.[17]

You've heard about the "eight glasses of water a day" thing, right? Well now that you're knocked up, it's ten. And if you're filling up on 16 ounces of liquid Lucifer at a time, chances are you're not getting your 80 ounces of water a day. Water is vital for detoxifying your body; it literally flushes out all the stored toxins. In addition, drinking a sufficient amount of water will prevent constipation. And preventing constipation will prevent the all-too-common pregnancy hemorrhoids. Water also transports nutrients from the food you eat to the baby. Aim for ten glasses a day—more if you're active. In the last trimester, especially, dehydration can lead to premature contractions and labor.[18] So drink up.

But stay away from the medicine cabinet! Maternal drug exposure has been said to cause at least ten percent of all birth defects.[19] Clinical trials for medicine are rarely performed on pregnant women. So we rely on trial and error, instead.[20] Some over-the-counter meds that seem to have had no ill side effects on fetuses are deemed "safe" for pregnant women. But perhaps if we took a closer look, we'd find alarming "coincidences." We just can't know for sure. What we do know is that in the first trimester, your baby's organs are developing. And medicine taken during this time can have an adverse effect on fetal development and cause birth defects and deformities. A severe enough birth defect can trigger miscarriage.[21] While the second trimester is considered "safest" for medicating, low birth weight and interference with nervous system development can result.[22] Third trimester medicating can trigger uterine contractions, causing early, delayed, or even prolonged labor. It can also limit baby's blood supply and cause complications after birth, like difficulty breathing. It is generally agreed upon that pregnant women should avoid aspirin, ibuprofen, and naproxen. Allergy meds can be made with aspirin, and many pain medicines contain aspirin, ibuprofen, or caffeine. So beware.[23] Some cough syrups and sleep aids contain alcohol. And even though heartburn is a common complaint, you're asking for trouble with antacids. Some contain sodium bicarbonate, which can cause constipation and gas and magnify water retention problems. Others have aluminum, which may also clog your butt and affect the way your body metabolizes other minerals. Excessive use of magnesium-based antacids can lead to magnesium poisoning.[24] Yes, experts have proclaimed Tylenol safe for pregnant women.[25] But use your own head. Do you think putting *chemicals* in your body is good for your unborn, developing fetus?

Usually, when we don't feel well, it is our body alerting us to the fact that something is wrong. And taking medicine doesn't necessarily cure the problem; it only masks the symptoms. So popping pills isn't the answer. Now, we know for some, the whole pregnancy experience can be taxing on the body. And at times, you may be uncomfortable or downright miserable. But do your best to suck it up. Think of it this way: Every ache and pain you endure without medicine prepares you for the ecstasy of squeezing an infant out of your V-spot. (Obviously, if you are on prescribed medication, you need to consult a physician before discontinuing it.)

We aren't trying to scare you with all this gloom and doom. We just want to give it to you straight. And if you can't take a little rough talk from two Skinny Bitches, then you aren't prepared to be a mother. 'Cause let's face it: kids can be little shits. So toughen up.

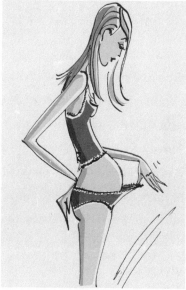

Chapter Two
Yes, It's Normal

O f course, you want this to be the best time of your whole life. But you've got these little nagging worries in the back of your mind keeping you from fully enjoying it. Obviously, it is important to see your doctor or midwife for anything that's troubling you. But let us put your mind at ease a little.

Your back hurts, huh? Bummer. But what you'd expect? You're carrying around extra weight. This shifts your center of gravity, which changes your posture. Also, your ligaments stretch and soften and your joints loosen to prepare you for labor.[26] Some women have backaches *and* sciatica, a sharp pain that can shoot all the way down to your heel. It totally sucks, but it's somewhat common—the uterus can press on the sciatic nerve. Back pain that's severe and unrelenting, low and dull, or accompanied by other symptoms should be brought to your doctor's attention.[27] But the other stuff just comes with the territory.

So does shortness of breath. Your uterus is expanding—shifting your organs, pressing on your diaphragm, and leaving your lungs with less room to expand. Also, you breathe more often, which can feel like shortness of breath.[28] Babies can really cramp your style, huh?

No, you don't have Chronic Fatigue Syndrome; it's normal to be tired throughout your pregnancy. Your hormone levels change rapidly in the first trimester, and there is an increase of progesterone, which can make you sleepy. Also, your body produces extra blood to help transport oxygen and nutrients to the fetus. This means more work for your heart and a greater demand on your entire circulatory system.[29] By the third trimester, your uterus is enlarged and you're carrying a baby inside it. Of course you're tired. Geesh.

But not too tired for sex, eh? Not only are your hormones raging (especially progesterone and estrogen) but you've also got increased blood flow to your boobs and your you-know-what. This can definitely lead to a higher sex drive. Plus, the fact that you aren't obsessing about getting pregnant anymore puts the fun back in sex. And you actually love your husband again, instead of just viewing him as a sperm donor. But if you want to kill him, that's normal, too. Many women are so sick during their first trimester—some throughout their entire pregnancies—that they have no libido at all. And let's face it: Lots of wives hate having sex anyway. (Note to husband: If you happen to read this, we didn't mean your wife. She loves sex.)

And he loves you, even though you're packing on the pounds. You're pregnant, and it's normal to gain weight. Now is not the time to be neurotic about your appearance or be obsessed with your favorite jeans. We only titled the book *Skinny Bitch: Bun in the Oven* to get your attention. Seriously. It was a sneaky marketing ploy. But the last thing a pregnant woman should be doing is worrying about her figure. Provided you aren't pigging out with reckless abandon, your weight gain will be justifiable and totally temporary.

Unless you're constipated and having trouble "dropping

the kids off at the pool." One of the important functions of pooping is weight maintenance. And unfortunately, constipation is a common side effect of pregnancy. All the hormonal changes—especially the increase in progesterone—affect the digestive process. Your colon is absorbing more water than usual, which can make your poops a little dryer and harder to come by. Gentle exercise can whip your ass and bowels into shape. The increase in oxygen can increase your intestinal action. And some workouts, like tai chi and yoga, can stimulate internal activity.[30] Good for your butt, good for your baby. But if you're still plagued by a brown blockade, you're probably not eating as well as you could. Avoid products that are highly processed and contain white flour, like most cookies, cakes, donuts, pastas, breads, and bagels. (If you're craving one, just ask yourself, "Am I willing to get hemorrhoids for *this*?") Also, up your fluid intake with water, juices, home-made soups, and fruit smoothies. And consider your anal issues as extra incentive to eat healthy, fibrous foods like fruits, vegetables, leafy greens, legumes, nuts, seeds, oatmeal, brown rice, and wholegrain breads and muffins.

Granted, you may be farting like a caveman and wary of adding fibrous fuel to the fire. But gas and pregnancy go hand in hand, so get over it. Avoid fried foods and other junk, for starters. And try to eat multiple small meals, instead of three jumbo ones. Really chew your food and eat slowly. You can also experiment with food combining. For example, try eating starchier foods (potatoes, brown rice, whole grains) with less starchy foods (leafy greens, broccoli, string beans). If your gas is actually *painful* (not just embarrassing or inconvenient), you can eliminate or reduce your intake of onions, garlic, legumes, and cabbage.[31] But these foods are healthy and shouldn't be avoided just to prevent a few toots. Sure it can be embarrassing, but personally, we think farting is almost as much fun as eating. Consider yourself lucky.

Unless you have heartburn, which totally sucks. Sorry. But it's very common, due again to those dastardly hormones, especially estrogen and progesterone. And the fact that your expanded uterus can shove your stomach out of its normal position doesn't help, either. Eating smaller, more frequent meals should help somewhat. So should drinking between meals, instead of during them. Try not to go to bed or lie down after overloading with food. And, as previously mentioned, abstain from coffee, alcohol, wine, beer, and fried foods. It's also a good idea to steer clear of spicy foods, carbonated drinks, rich pastries, and more than a tad bit of chocolate. Especially since excessive weight gain can cause heartburn. Since misery loves company, take comfort in knowing that as many as 80 percent of pregnant women are in heartburn hell, too.[32] Some women have it all the way through, but generally it sucks in the fifth month and blows in the final three. If you are immobilized by it, consult with an herbalist or naturopath for herbal remedies. But first try some chamomile tea.

But don't expect to find a quick fix for your mood swings. There are thirty different hormones present in your body during pregnancy! And in the last trimester, your prolactin level increases to stimulate milk production. So the third trimester can be extra hairy. Just resign yourself to feeling crazy, weepy, or ready to kill someone for nine months. That way, you'll be prepared for the worst, but pleasantly surprised if you keep it together.

We cannot emphasize enough the importance of a healthy, well-balanced diet for warding off mood swings. For starters, be sure to get an adequate amount of vitamins through your diet. Popping a pill once a day isn't nearly as effectual as what you're eating throughout the day. Literally, a single meal can affect your mood and make or break your whole day. Foods rich in B vitamins jack up your levels of dopamine and serotonin, your "feel good" neurotransmitters. So load up on apricots, avocados, bananas, dates, figs, lentils, lima beans, soybeans, peanuts, pumpkin seeds, almonds (raw), sesame seeds, walnuts, green leafy vegetables, brewer's yeast, tofu, spirulina, and whole grains (like brown rice, buckwheat, oats, millet, quinoa, and wheat germ). (We realize that some of these foods may seem unappetizing if you're not used to them, but they'll grow on you.) These foods are also rich in carbohydrates, which can completely affect your state of mind.

Ever wonder why you crave sugar (carbs) or comfort food (carbs) when you're depressed? It's like this: eating carbs causes a release of insulin, which, in turn, creates a temporary reduction of all your amino acid levels except tryptophan. Without competition from the other aminos, your tryptopahn levels increase. And tryptophan gets converted into serotonin, a "feel good" neurotransmitter. So eating carbs is your body's way of self-medicating. Which is totally fine, provided you're eating healthy complex carbs and not refined sugar, white flour, white bread, white rice, regular pasta, or other highly processed foods. These simple carbs spike your "feel good" levels and then send them crashing down, which can make you feel moody, irritable, tired, depressed, absent-minded, lethargic, or insane.

High protein diets can have similar negative effects by reducing levels of serotonin and tryptophan.[33] So pay attention to your carb intake. Even with the good carbs, notice how you feel immediately after or a short while later. If they make you feel sleepy or mopey, eat your day's largest portion at dinnertime, instead of in the middle of the day. That way, you can take your cranky ass to bed instead of walking around miserable all day. But don't avoid carbs altogether. They are super important for you and your baby, and you should have complex carb rations with every meal.

Again, eating several small meals throughout the day, as opposed to three big ones, is a helpful tool. And again, caffeine and sugar should be avoided. These two punks can totally sabotage your moods and cause depression and fatigue. Another weapon in your arsenal against mood swings: exercise. When we exercise, our brains release endorphins and other "feel good" opiates. So if you're battling your emotions, get active and see if it helps. (Yoga is great for physical exercise and emotional release.)

All the while, never underestimate the power of friendship. Talk out your problems. Confess your fears. Share your demons. Often, a dose of good friends can ease the biggest burdens. If that doesn't work, try a dose of peppermint, spearmint, or raspberry tea (caffeine-free, of course).

If you're avoiding bad foods, eating healthy ones, exercising regularly, having regular powwows, but still feeling depressed—Get help. There is no shame in saying, "This isn't right. I'm taking excellent care of myself and doing all the right things, but I still feel crummy. I need help." Keep your doctor apprised of the situation, but try a naturopath and/or herbalist. If that doesn't do the trick, visit your doctor and investigate your options. While we fully promote natural remedies and believe that most problems can be treated holistically, we know that in some instances, traditional medical treatments are needed.

It's not bad enough you're losing all your marbles, but now you've gotta lose your lunch, too? Morning sickness can be a real bitch. And not just in the morning, either. It's estimated that 50–85 percent of all pregnant women suffer from this puke-fest, especially during the first trimester. But rest assured, it usually ends around twelve to sixteen weeks. There are many theories regarding the cause of morning sickness: One hypothesis is that your body is adjusting to all the hormonal changes. Another suggests an increased sensitivity to odors. Or it could be that while progesterone relaxes the muscles in the uterus to prevent early labor, it also relaxes the stomach and intestines, causing excess stomach acids. Some claim morning sickness is an evolutionary adaptation that keeps pregnant women away from foods that may harm their developing fetuses. (Interesting concept, since the foods that most commonly repulse women in the first trimester are the most likely to carry harmful parasites: meat, poultry, eggs, and fish.) Stress, a vitamin B-6 deficiency, low blood sugar levels, or chemical by-products of the increased hormones have also been blamed. Maybe. Maybe. Maybe. Or maybe it's due to HCG (human chorionic gonadotrophin), the increased hormone that shows up in positive pregnancy tests.[34]

Whatever the reason for morning sickness, it sucks. But there are as many suggested remedies as there are theories. And while we hate to sound like a broken record, eating smaller, frequent meals might help. As can eating complex carbs while avoiding caffeine; sugar; and spicy, fried, and rich foods. Many women swear by crackers, which we're happy to endorse, so long as they're made from whole grains and not white or bleached flour. (Also make sure they don't contain sugar, corn syrup, or hydrogenated oils.) Some women tout vitamin B-6 and up their intake by eating bananas, brown rice, corn, nuts, whole grains, avocados, and potatoes, or they take supplements. Others drink chamomile, raspberry, fennel seed, ginger, peppermint, spearmint, or anise tea (all caffeine-free). A cup of tea may do the trick, but don't overdose on it, because it can cause uterine stimulation. You're just going to have to experiment until you find something that works for you. Just do your best to replenish your fluids throughout the day, as constant puking will dehydrate you.

And don't shit your drawers if you notice a little blood in them. A week to ten days after conception, implantation bleeding can occur when the fertilized egg attaches to the uterine wall. And it's estimated that one in five women experience spotting during their first trimester. Some even have light bleeding for the first six months, occurring when their menstrual cycle would've taken place.[35] Weird, huh? Certainly, it's alarming to see blood in your undies when you're pregnant. And in some cases, it could be a problem. But it's also very common. So do not panic and immediately go to your dark place of "Something's wrong. I'm having a miscarriage. It's because I was a slut in college." Try to remain calm (and optimistic) and call your doctor or midwife.

She'll also be able to allay your fears about that itching down south. No, your baby didn't give you crabs. (Although you should check with your gyno to make sure you didn't get an STD during your slutty college days.) Yeast infections are common during pregnancy and can result from either the high level of pregnancy hormones or a pH imbalance.[36] Regardless of the cause, you'll likely be converted into a crotch-scratching lunatic. Embarrassing, but normal.

Oh yeah, so is that sludge in your underwear. It's just a cocktail of normal bacterial flora and old cells shed from the walls of your VJ. It's the same snail trail that was in your pants before you got pregnant, there's just more of it now due to the increase in hormones and greater blood flow to your cookie.[37]

And lots of grown women piss their pants. Nothing to be ashamed of. Again, all your organs are getting moved around and pressed on. The pressure on your bladder can cause a little leakage throughout the day. Ha ha.

It's also likely that you'll have to pee more. Your body has about 30–50 percent more blood than it did before. This means your kidneys are working harder to filter the increase in blood, which means more sissy.[38]

Which normally wouldn't be so bad, but your legs and ankles are the size of tree trunks. The swelling is perfectly normal. It's caused by the increase of all the extra fluids in your body. (A sudden swelling of your hands and face, however, is *not* normal! That could signify preeclampsia—call your doctor ASAP!)[39]

So your back's killing you, you've got heartburn *and* cankles, your bladder's leaking, and your cooch is itching like crazy. All you want is a good night's sleep after another full day of torture. Only you can't get @%#* comfortable, because you you've got gas, shortness of breath, and you have to get up every two minutes to pee. As your pregnancy progresses, it also becomes harder to find a comfortable position to sleep. Mother Nature isn't cruel. She's just preparing you for the sleepless nights to come.

Ah, the joys of motherhood.

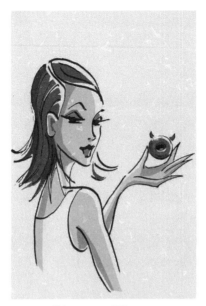

Chapter Three
Sugar Is Satan

Now, we know we mentioned earlier that sugar was bad news for morning sickness and mood swings. We were sugarcoating it then. The real truth: Sugar totally sucks for you and your baby. Just when you thought you could pig out unabashedly. . . . Sorry. We know it's devastating news.

To reiterate and expand—sugar has a detrimental effect on mood swings. It enters the bloodstream like gangbusters—hard and fast. It causes blood sugar levels to spike, then crash.

This crash can leave you feeling tired, depressed, or cranky. Now, you may be thinking, "Who cares? I'll risk feeling crummy for a few hours." Unfortunately, sugar is like crack, and eating it is like opening Pandora's box. When your body starts to crash, it attempts to maintain balance by creating a craving. A craving for what? More sugar, duh.[40] Adding frequent sugar crashes to your already fluctuating hormones ... you might as well check yourself into an asylum until the baby comes.

And when you get out, check yourself into a fat farm. 'Cause sugar will make you fat. Excess amounts of sugar are stored in the liver as glycogen. But when the liver is too full, those excess amounts are returned to the bloodstream as fatty acids.[41] If you are in your second or third trimester, you need to be eating 200 to 300 extra calories every day. But if they're coming from sugar, then they're empty calories. Meaning, they're a total waste. You'll be packing on the pounds, but neither you or baby will be getting any nutrients. There's nothing nutritional or beneficial in refined, processed sugar. Which is why you'll never feel satisfied after eating it, and you'll just want to eat more, more, more.

We know that pregnancy can be stressful at times, and we

know that stress can cause us to eat crap. Especially in the form of sugar. (Hell, even when we're not stressed, we Americans eat our weight in sugar every year.)[42] But it's vital to find ways to cope with stress that aren't harmful. When we eat foods high in sugar, we're usually also getting large amounts of fat. And a high intake of sugar and fat increases the risk of preeclampsia.[43] (Preeclampsia can lead to high blood pressure, kidney drama, seizures, and convulsions.) Kinda makes that Twinkie a little less appealing, huh?

How'd you like to have a bunch of annoying, little colds throughout your pregnancy? Studies show that eating sugar causes a decrease in white blood cell counts. And white blood cells are our first line of defense against illness. So eating sugar compromises your immune system, leaving you and your baby susceptible to colds, the flu, and all sorts of other trouble.[44]

What sorts of other trouble? Here's a little biology lesson: When we eat, most of our food is broken down into glucose (a kind of sugar), which will provide us with energy. The glucose enters the bloodstream. And when everything is functioning well, the pancreas produces insulin, which allows the glucose to enter the liver, muscles, and fatty tissue.[45] But sometimes, the pancreas doesn't produce enough insulin, and the glucose remains in the bloodstream. This elevated level of glucose in the blood is called *diabetes*.

Pregnancy hormones make it harder for the body to utilize insulin. So in most cases, the pancreas will simply secrete more. But on occasion, the pancreas can't keep up with the body's demand for insulin. This results in gestational diabetes. Even though it only affects two to seven percent of expectant moms, it's one of the most common pregnancy health problems.[46]

One concern with gestational diabetes is that high blood sugar levels can cause macrosomia, or an excessively large baby. This means the baby could be too big to enter the birth canal. Or that the baby's head will enter, but then his or her shoulders will get stuck.[47] Of course, this can be resolved by having a C-section. But even after delivery, the baby's not out of the water. Babies born to moms with gestational diabetes have a higher risk of hypoglycemia (low blood sugar), hypocalcemia (low calcium in the blood), polycythemia (an increase in red blood cells), and jaundice.[48]

Even if they dodge those bullets, there is a higher likelihood that later in life they can develop diabetes or suffer from childhood or adult obesity.[49] Happy birthday! I got you dia-

betes and a lifetime of weight problems! I also increased the
risk for you to be born with respiratory distress syndrome and
heart abnormalities.[50] Compared with those with normal
blood sugar levels, pregnant women with uncontrolled
diabetes are three times more likely to have babies with mal-
formed hearts.[51]

We aren't trying to give you nightmares about twenty-pound
babies with rectangular-shaped hearts. When detected, gestational diabetes can be managed. So if you are diagnosed, don't
despair. We just want you to do all you can to avoid these risks.
And by that, we mean eating really well, staying away from
sugar, and exercising (unless your doctor says you can't).
Studies show that moderate exercise helps keep blood sugar
levels controlled.[52]

Gestational diabetes not only affects you *now*, but it affects
your future, as well. About two-thirds of women who get
gestational diabetes wind up getting it again during future
pregnancies. Also, studies show that approximately 50 percent of women with gestational diabetes wind up developing
type II diabetes within five years of giving birth.[53] Congratulations! You're a mom! And a diabetic!

Sugar isn't just the diabetes devil. It can do a lot of other damage, too. Everyone knows that sugar can cause gum disease and tooth decay. But most people don't know it can also lead to glycation—when sugar molecules abnormally attach to cells in the body—causing an acceleration in aging to the eyes, brain, and nervous system. Maybe that's a good thing; you won't be able to see or feel that it's also causing saggy skin, poor organ function, and arterial stiffness.[54] Not turned off yet? Refined sugar has also been linked to yeast overgrowth (check your undies), hyperactivity, attention deficit disorder, enlargement of the liver and kidneys, mental and emotional disorders, and an imbalance of neurotransmitters in the brain.[55] Yikes!

We know, in a sense, we're ruining your life, delivering all this bad news about sugar. You just wanted to read a light, fluffy, "how-to-eat when you're pregnant" book, and now we've gone and taken away your greatest joy. We're truly sorry. But we warned you in the Bitchclaimer. Here it is again, if you forgot:

"We didn't write this book to make friends. We wrote this book to help women eat right, ensuring successful pregnancies and healthy babies. So if you want to hear "everything in moderation," "an occasional glass of wine is fine," or any other

candy-coated bullshit, pick another book. Skinny Bitch: Bun in the Oven *will tell you the truth about food and how what you eat affects your pregnancy and baby.*

"Go make friends at your Lamaze classes. We're invested in making a difference in your life."

We're not just committed to healthy pregnancies and babies. We truly want you to continue to take care of yourself after you give birth and for the rest of your life. We want you to adopt a healthier lifestyle now and pass it on to your children. We genuinely care. So with that said, unfortunately, we have more bad news.

Refined sugar isn't the only sweetener that sucks. High fructose corn syrup (HFCS) blows, too. When you ingest natural sugars (like those found in fruits or whole grains), your brain signals to your body that it's satisfied and that you don't need to eat any more. With HFCS, this doesn't occur. So high intakes of HFCS can lead to obesity, which increases your risk of type II diabetes and heart disease. Our livers don't metabolize HFCS the same way they do other sugars. HFCS can increase the blood level of triglycerides (bad fats that clog arteries and cause cardiovascular disease).[56] It's hard to find information on how HFCS affects developing fetuses. But the fact that it's so bad for our bodies leads us to believe it's doubly bad for developing babies. And unfortunately, because HFCS is so cheap to produce, food manufacturers love it and put it in almost everything. Check your pantries, refrigerators, and freezers. Then throw all the shit away!

While you're at it, get rid of your Sweet 'N Low, too, since saccharin (found in Sweet 'N Low) can easily cross the placenta and enter the fetal bloodstream.[57] It's believed that an accumulation of saccharin can cause bladder cancer to the fetus.[58]

And artificial sweeteners made with aspartame, like NutraSweet and Equal, might be even more sinister than sugar and HFCS combined. So many people have been sickened by this shit that there are aspartame victim support groups. Some of the ninety-two aspartame side effects listed by the Food and Drug Administration (FDA) include memory loss, nerve cell damage, migraines, brain lesions, joint pain, Alzheimer's, bloating, nervous system disorders, hair loss, food cravings, weight gain, and reproductive disorders.[59]

So how the hell did this poison get FDA approval? Well, where there's a will ($), there's a way. And in the case of aspartame, former Senator Howard Metzenbaum said it "was approved by the FDA in circumstances that can only be described as troubling."[60]

He could've been referring to any number of things:

- When founder G.D. Searle put aspartame before the FDA for approval, it was denied *eight* times. In 1975, the FDA put together a task force to review Searle's testing methods. Task force team leader Phillip Brodsky said he "had never seen anything as bad as Searle's testing" and called the test results "manipulated."[61]

- One FDA statistician called data on aspartame "worrisome." An FDA toxicologist testified before Congress that aspartame could cause brain tumors.[62]

- In 1977, the FDA asked the U.S. attorney's office to start grand jury proceedings against Searle for "knowingly misrepresenting findings and concealing material facts and making false statements in aspartame safety tests." Shortly after, the U.S. attorney leading the investigation against Searle was offered a job by the law firm that was representing Searle. Later that same year, he resigned as the U.S. attorney and withdrew from the case, delaying the grand jury's investigation. This caused the statute of limitations on the charges to run out, and the investigation was dropped. And he accepted the job with Searle's law firm![63]

- In 1980, a review by the Public Board of Inquiry set up by the

FDA determined that aspartame should not be approved. The board said it had "not been presented with proof of reasonable certainty that aspartame is safe for use as a food additive." In 1981, a new FDA Commissioner was appointed. Despite the fact that three out of six scientists advised against approval, the commissioner decided to overrule the scientific review panel and allow aspartame into limited dry goods. In 1983, he got it approved for beverages even though the National Soft Drink Association urged the FDA to delay approval until further testing could be done. That same year, the commissioner left the FDA amid charges of impropriety. The Internal Department of Health and Human Services was investigating him for accepting gratuities from FDA-regulated companies. He went to work as a consultant for Searle's public relations firm![64]

- The FDA finally urged Congress to prosecute Searle for giving the government false or incomplete test results on aspartame. However, the two government attorneys assigned to the case decided not to prosecute. Later, they went to work for the law firm that represented Searle![65]

- In 1996, the FDA approved aspartame for use without restrictions.[66]

• A study funded by Monsanto (the company that owned NutraSweet) was conducted to see if there were possible birth defects associated with consuming aspartame. After preliminary data revealed damaging information, the study was cut off.[67]

(Did we mention that aspartame is a *billion* dollar industry?[68])

Dr. John Olney is a neuropathologist, neuroscientist, and a world expert on excitotoxicity. (In layman's terms, excitotoxicity is when brain cells get "excited" to death.) Dr. Olney's own lab studies demonstrated that aspartame could cause excitotoxicity. Using the existing data of other scientists, he also published a study reporting a 65 percent increase in human brain tumors since the FDA approved aspartame.[69]

When methyl alcohol, a component of aspartame, enters the body, it turns into formaldehyde. Formaldehyde is toxic and carcinogenic (cancer-causing).[70] Studies conducted at the University of Barcelona revealed that formaldehyde causes breaks in DNA. Men and women who consume aspartame can have breaks in their sperm and egg DNA. This can increase risks of cancer and developmental problems in their offspring.[71] (So your husband needs to get off the junk, too!)

Former neurosurgeon Dr. Russell Blaylock is one of the

world's foremost authorities on the biochemistry of aspartame and its effect on brain function. He states quite clearly that "pregnant women should never consume foods containing aspartame.... The aspartic acid, phenylalanine, and methanol [components of aspartame] are all known to produce abnormal development of a baby's brain."[72]

Also regarded as one of the foremost "aspartamologists," three-time Pulitzer Prize nominee[73] Dr. H. J. Roberts is vehemently opposed, as well. "Having been involved in medical practice, teaching, and the authorship of texts for a half a century, I do not casually make statements that might jeopardize a longstanding reputation...."[74] I continue to urge ALL pregnant women and mothers who breast-feed to avoid aspartame products.... The manifestation of aspartame disease in young children include severe headache, convulsions, unexplained vision loss, rashes, asthma, gastrointestinal problems, obesity, marked weight loss, hypoglycemia, diabetes, addiction (probably largely due to the methyl alcohol), hyperthyroidism, and a host of neuropsychiatric features [including] extreme fatigue, irritability, hyperactivity, depression, antisocial behavior (including suicide), poor school performance, the deterioration of intelligence, and brain tumors."[75] Hmm . . .

have a diet soda that will last fifteen minutes or have a fucked up kid that will last a lifetime? Tough decision.

Despite all the drama and trauma related to aspartame, more than two-thirds of adults in our society consume it in some form. Approximately 40 percent of children do, as well.[76]

Many nutritionists and healthcare providers think aspartame is safe because it's composed of two amino acids (phenylalanine and aspartic acid) that are also found in protein foods. However, protein foods have more than just the two amino acids found in aspartame. The other amino acids serve as "neutralizers." So when you're ingesting aspartame, your bloodstream is getting "flooded" with the two amino acids. Taking the two amino acids out of their natural state is like taking words out of context.[77] Bad news bears.

Chances are, your ob/gyn will tell you it's fine to consume aspartame in moderate doses unless you have the genetic disorder phenylketonuria (PKU). (People with PKU can't metabolize phenylalanine.)[78] So if your doctor says aspartame is okay in moderate doses, does that mean you should consume it? No! Get your head out of your ass. Smarten up. Get off the diet soda, chewing gum, and all the other crap that contains aspartame. And never look back.

So no refined sugar, no Sweet 'N Low, no NutraSweet, and no Equal. We can already hear you diet soda junkies clucking away: "But what about Splenda?" "Is Splenda okay?" Hell to the no! Splenda's sly marketing slogan is, "made from sugar so it tastes like sugar." This is how they get us to think, "Hey, it's natural. It's made from sugar." But Splenda is about as natural as a breast implant filled with soybean oil. It's made by altering the molecular structure of sugar![79] Sucralose, the end result, is like Franken-sugar. The reason Splenda's touted as being zero calories is because the body can't even metabolize it![80] And the FDA approval process surrounding Splenda is even more McShady than the hijinks surrounding aspartame. Only two human trials were completed and published before the FDA deemed sucralose safe![81] Two! It gets worse. You may want to sit down. The two trials *combined* consisted of a mere thirty-six people, with only twenty-three actually given the product![82] Wait. Not done. The trial only lasted four friggin' days![83] Four days! Wait. There's more. The study only examined sucralose's effect on friggin' tooth decay![84] *After* FDA approval, Splenda conducted a "long-term" human toxicity study. For three months.[85] Three months?! What, are consumers only going to buy Splenda products for three

months, and then stop? Where we're from—Earth—that's
the biggest pile of steaming bullshit ever! So, is Splenda safe
to consume during your pregnancy? Couldn't tell ya. It wasn't
one of the few, pathetic, sham studies they conducted.[86]

If you aren't thoroughly turned off refined sugar and artificial sweeteners by now, you're a jackass. This is our last
attempt to get you off the crack pipe: Surely you've seen those
stupid deodorant commercials, "Strong enough for a man,
but pH balanced for a woman," right? Well, we have no idea
what the hell they're talking about. But we do know that
everything we eat has its own pH balance. When food is
digested, it leaves an acid or alkaline "ash" in the body,
depending on the food's mineral content. Surprise, surprise:
Refined sugars and artificial sweeteners are acid forming.[87]
(So are coffee—both regular and decaf—and other foods that
we'll get to later.) When our bodies get too acidic, we're much
more prone to illness. It can be something minor, like skin
problems, allergies, headaches, colds, or yeast infections. Or,
we can experience major trauma—severe damage to the thyroid gland, liver, and adrenal glands. Also, if our bodies
become too acidic, they'll withdraw minerals from our bones
and muscles.[88] Ever hear of osteoporosis? Keep gorging on

the refined sugar and artificial sweeteners and you'll be a bag of bones in no time. That is if cancer doesn't get you first; cancer cells thrive in acidic environments.[89] Last bit of bad news: Acidic foods cause your body to produce fat cells, in order to keep acid away from your organs.[90]

(Now, logically, you would think that citrus fruits are acidic, but actually, when they enter the body, they are alkalizing. They contain potassium and calcium, which are alkalizing minerals. They also have a high percentage of alkaline salts. Nearly all fruits, vegetables, and legumes are alkaline when they enter the body.)[91]

We know this is a lot to swallow. And if you're outraged at the FDA and companies who profit off poisoning us—good. You should be. But don't sit there stewing in hate and rage. Not good for the baby. Get off your arse, clean out your kitchen, and throw all that shit in the trash. And don't be mad at us! We had to tell you.

And it may sound impossible and unbelievable now, but you *can* kick the sugar/artificial sweetener habit. And if you do, you'll really get a sense of how shitty the stuff makes you feel if you try eating it again after going a while without it.

We realize it's a tall order, and that for some people, death would be a better option than giving up sweets. If you're of that ilk, there are some ways to help curb your sweet tooth. For starters, drink water. Many times, a glass of water will erase a craving. It sounds lame, but it works. Another trick is simply waiting out the craving. Studies have shown that if you wait fifteen to thirty minutes, the desire to eat junk will pass. So get up, go for a walk, make a phone call, work on your nursery, do something to busy yourself. You may forget all about the donut. If that doesn't work, brush your teeth. There's nothing like clean teeth and fresh, minty breath to make junk food less appealing. Or have a cup of decaf peppermint tea; it comes across as sweet in a confusing way. (FYI: These little ploys work for all junk food, not just sugar.)

But if you gotta have something sweet, eat something sweet. Hold on—don't get too excited. Fruit. We're talking about fruit. Fruit is sweet. And it's good for you and baby. As pathetic and miserable as it sounds, you'll be astounded by this little caper. Fruit totally squelches sugar cravings. Try it a few times before you go pissing all over it.

If you tried all the above and you're still dying for something sweet, eat something sweet for crying out loud. (*Now* you can get excited.) Food is our passion, and we never want to feel deprived. So when we want something sweet, we eat it. We just don't eat our old, standard crap with sugar, high fructose corn syrup, or artificial sweeteners. The following substitutes are less processed than regular sugar and less hazardous than corn syrup and artificial sweeteners: evaporated cane juice, Sucanat, brown rice syrup, barley malt syrup, Rapadura sugar, Turbinado sugar, raw sugar, beet sugar, date sugar, maple syrup, molasses, blackstrap molasses, and agave nectar.[92] So **read the ingredients** of the junk food you want, and only eat the ones that have these sweeteners. But don't gorge yourself on any one of them. A few little nibbles can quash the sweet tooth urge. If they don't, it's because you're hungry *and* you're having a sweet craving. Address the hunger first. Then have the little sweet. Don't be havin' no binge-athon with a box of Ring Dings.

"Read the ingredients." We're going to be saying this a lot. And the reason is simple: You should care about what you're putting in your body. At the very least, you should know what you're putting in your body. So from now on, read the ingredients of every single thing you buy. And use your head. If you're buying juice, there's no reason it should have sweetener of any kind in it. It's fruit—it's already sweet! If you're buying healthy foods, there shouldn't be sweeteners in them—sweeteners are for desserts, not meals! If you're buying soda, you're an asshole because we've already told you how terrible it is for your body and your baby. If you're buying junk food, it shouldn't have sugar, corn syrup, or artificial sweeteners. Got it? (We know it's a lot to take in, so in chapter eight, we give you an acceptable junk food list, chock-full of cookies, chips, ice cream, and other goodies! We just didn't put it in this chapter because there are a few other things we wanted to teach you first. It's hard work organizing a book!)

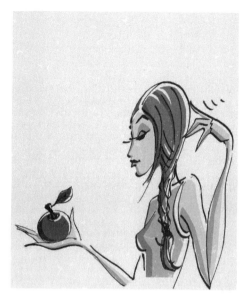

Chapter Four
Carbs: Eat 'Em, Dumb-Ass

Unless you spent the last few years under a rock, you've heard all the "low-carb" hype. Unless you're as dumb as a box of rocks, you'll ignore it. There is a small portion of the trend that's actually sensible. The rest is bunk.

There are two types of carbs: simple and complex. To remember which is which, think "simple=shitty." Simple, shitty carbs are the ones you want to avoid, clearly. They have little to no nutritional value, are highly processed and refined, and totally suck for your body and your baby. They're made up mostly of sugar, which releases too quickly, almost violently, into our bodies, causing "sugar highs" and then "crashes." This tends to leave us hungry, so we eat more. Simple carbs include soda, candy, white breads, white rice, white flour, white pasta (durum semolina), sugar, and most refined, processed foods. These are the bad boys that gave all carbs a bad reputation.

For some asinine reason, food manufacturers decided that we wouldn't buy their products unless they were white and soft. So they took natural grains, like brown rice and whole wheat, and stripped away all their nutrients, vitamins, and minerals to achieve the color and texture change. This refining process totally compromises the nutritional integrity of the food—all for appearances. So companies then add these nutrients back into their refined, milled foods and use terms like "enriched" or "fortified." But there's no use trying to fool with Mother Nature. Our bodies cannot absorb these added-in minerals with the same ease.[93] Tragically, most cereals, pastas, rice, bagels, breads, cookies, muffins, cakes, and pastries have been bastardized in this manner. Pay attention to how your body feels when you eat these foods. Chances are you'll notice moderate to severe mood swings and energy surges and losses. The only sensible suggestion made by low-carb diets is to avoid these shitty, simple carbs.

But all carbs aren't created equal. Complex carbs are not only good for you, they're vital. And unlike simple carbs, complex carbs release gradually, providing a steady source of energy. Avoiding or limiting them, as suggested by low-carb diets, is stupid, senseless, and dangerous. Before you got pregnant, complex carbs should've been the majority of your diet. If they weren't before, they definitely should be now. Carbs are the body's main source of energy. Even though fat and protein can be burned for fuel, carbs are the most efficient energy source.[94] And they're loaded with vitamins, minerals, phytochemicals, and other essential nutrients.[95] They also have a shitload of fiber, which is good for, well, shitting. Complex carbs are fruits, vegetables, whole grains, nuts, seeds, and legumes (beans, lentils).

To be clear, yes, we said "fruit." Eat it. The most irritating thing about the low-carb craze is the resistance to eating fruit. Fruit is, quite possibly, the most perfect food in existence. It is unique in that it barely requires any work to be digested. High in enzymes, it effortlessly passes through the body, supplying carbohydrates, fiber, vitamins, minerals, fatty acids, amino acids, and cancer-fighting tannins and flavonoids. Because it is made up of mostly water, fruit hydrates the body and aids in cleansing, detoxifying, and eliminating. There is nothing more irritating than some jackass woman announcing she doesn't eat fruit because it's "too high in sugar." Or that she doesn't drink juice because "it has too many calories." Get a clue. Start thinking for yourself for one second. If you do, you'll realize that fruit is God's gift to us all. And it's a carb.

Lots of times when you think you're having a satanic sugar craving, it's actually a carb craving. And brushing your teeth or taking a walk won't make it go away. And you shouldn't try to make it go away. Complex carbs are good for you! And for your moods! We often unknowingly try to regulate our moods with food. Eating complex carbs has a positive effect on our serotonin (feel-good neurotransmitters) levels. (Conversely, eating a high-protein diet can have a negative effect on serotonin levels.)[96] So when you're feeling tired, cranky, or depressed, instead of eating a piece of cake, eat an apple or a piece of wholegrain toast and feel human again.

Seriously, it's really important you don't deny yourself complex carbs during your pregnancy. If you do, your body will start using fat and protein for energy, which can impede the development of the baby's brain and nervous system. Burning fat releases ketones (acid by-product), which can destroy fetal brain cells and can negatively affect the baby's pH balance, making it too acidic.[97] Keto-acidosis can lower fetal blood pressure and raise fetal heart rate.[98] Not only can ketones affect your baby's pH, but they can also cause yours to be too acidic and can make you dehydrated and constipated.[99] (P.S. It'll also make you smell like a bag of ass.)

So you have hemorrhoids from lack of fiber, your baby's a dumb-dumb, and you're weak from dehydration. All because you read some stupid book or bought into the low-carb hype. Pitiful. Please, for the sake of your pregnancy and health of your baby, eat fruits, vegetables, whole grains, nuts, seeds, and legumes. They are complex carbohydrates and they provide energy, vitamins, minerals, and are directly responsible for fueling fetal cell division (meaning they actually help *make* your baby).[100]

Shitty, simple carbs—bad. Avoid 'em. Complex carbs—good. Eat 'em.

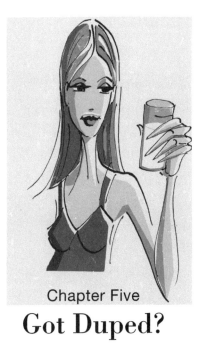

Chapter Five

Got Duped?

BLIND OBEDIENCE

In the 1960s, Yale University psychologist Stanley Milgram conducted an experiment to prove the theory of blind obedience. Participants were led to believe that the study would examine the effect punishment has on learning. For this purpose, they were asked to deliver electric shocks to another participant, The Subject (whom they couldn't see), whenever The Subject answered a question incorrectly. What the participants didn't know was that *they* were the ones being studied and that The Subjects were hired actors and there was no electric shock actually being delivered. To Milgram's surprise, the majority of participants "shocked" another human simply because they were told to do so, even though it made them uncomfortable and even though The Subject could be heard screaming through the wall. More alarming is that 61–66 percent of participants were willing to deliver a fatal shock![101] Blind obedience.

Why are we telling you about The Milgram Experiment in a "how-to-eat" guide for pregnant women? Because we all suffer from blind obedience in some form or another at one time or another. We do what we're told. We're part of the masses. We go with the grain. We read something in a magazine or see it on the news, and it becomes gospel.

There are countless studies on every topic. But all too often, the studies are funded by groups who stand to profit from them. As a result, the findings are sometimes skewed. Regardless, many findings are considered the end all, be all, and they have been widely accepted by the entire population to be true. News is reported, and in the blink of an eye, millions of us accept it as truth. Not only that, but we tell millions more. Now this "truth" is floating around in the universe, and we all believe it as strongly as if we had conducted the study ourselves. Think about it. In how many ways do you advise people using "facts" you "know to be true," simply because you have heard them being said for years? These "facts" become ingrained in our personal "truths," and we pass them out as if they were our own. And the cycle never ends. "Ginger ale is good for an upset stomach." "Black coffee sobers you up." "You need milk for strong bones." The truth: *Ginger root* is good for an upset stomach. But most sodas have artificial flavors, and no ginger at all. (And the ones that do have ginger have it in such small amounts, it's insignificant.) Coffee can make you alert, but it sure as hell ain't gonna make you sober. And as for milk and osteoporosis . . . um, this chapter will likely send your whole world crashing down.

And your first instinct will be to not believe what we're saying. Because admitting your whole life has been based on an enormous lie is a jagged pill to swallow. It'd be much easier to toss this book aside, call us "crazy bitches," and go on your way. Easy as it would be, we don't think you'll do that. We have faith in you. We know you can think for yourself and keep an open mind. We know that you want to. And we know that because you care about your temple and your baby growing inside it, the truth is paramount to you.

Brace yourselves. Here it is: There is no reason on earth that pregnant women should be drinking cows' milk. For that matter, no adult humans should be drinking cows' milk. Forget everything you've ever learned about dairy for a minute and try to approach it from a fresh perspective.

COMMON SENSE, BITCHES

Think about it: When a woman gives birth, she produces milk and breastfeeds her baby. When the baby reaches a certain age, the mother weans him or her off breast milk and feeds the baby solid food. After the mother's milk dries up, the child never drinks her breast milk ever again. Cows (and every other mammal on the planet) are exactly the same. Contrary to popular belief, cows do not need to be milked. They have udders, just like women have breasts, even when they aren't lactating. They only produce milk when they give birth. And like humans and every other mammal on the planet, cows nurse their young, wean them, and then never provide them with milk ever again. This is where our similarities end. Human beings are the only species on the entire planet that drinks milk as adults. And we're the only species on the planet that drinks the milk of another species.

Did you ever stop to really think about why? Probably not. Why would you? We've all been told our entire lives that we need cows' milk for calcium. That without milk, we won't grow big and strong and that without milk, our bones and teeth will crumble. Our parents, teachers, doctors—everyone told us milk was an absolute necessity. So it never occurred to us to question it. So again, forgetting everything you've learned about why you "need" milk, think about it. Why on earth would Mother Nature require human beings to drink the milk of another species after we've stopped drinking our own mothers' breast milk? Why would we "need" to get calcium from the milk of another species after being weaned from our own kind? The answer: We don't.

BONE LOSS, CANCER, AND ILLNESS, OH MY!

The Harvard Nurses' Health Study followed more than 75,000 women over the course of twelve years. And guess what? **Milk was not shown to have a protective effect on bones.** In fact, quite the contrary. **The study revealed that dairy products were associated with an increased risk of fractures.** [102] Researchers at Yale did a study using thirty-four surveys from sixteen countries found in twenty-nine research publications. They reported the same findings.[103] Americans are among the top consumers of dairy products in the world. So if dairy does what the dairy industry claims, we should have among the lowest rates of osteoporosis in the world, right? According to *The Journal of Gerontology*, American women over fifty have among the highest rates of hip fractures in the world. The only countries with higher rates are those that consume more milk![104] If you're not outraged, you aren't paying attention. The whole reason we douse ourselves with dairy is because it "strengthens bones." But scientific studies show that it does the exact opposite! If you aren't seething mad right now, check your pulse. You've been living a lie your whole life so that a few people could make money! (P.S. Consuming high amounts of dairy blocks iron absorption, contributing to iron deficiency.)[105]

Cows' milk has one of the lowest absorption rates of all calcium sources.[106] One reason is its high protein content. A study showed vegans (people who abstain from animal products, including dairy) and omnivores having the same blood levels of calcium, even though the omnivores ingested *twice as much calcium*.[107] Yes, milk is high in calcium, but it's not an efficient source for it. Remember in chapter three when we talked about how sugar creates an acidic environment in the body? Well, so do dairy products. And this acidity causes an excretion of calcium in the urine.[108] Loss of calcium . . . osteoporosis.

Remember from chapter three what else an acidic environment causes? Ca-ca-ca-cancer. Ovarian cancer is just one cancer that has been linked to dairy consumption. A Harvard study found that when women with low enzyme levels consumed dairy on a regular basis, their risk of ovarian cancer was up to *three times* greater.[109] Are you pissed *now*?

And according to *The China Study*'s Dr. T. Colin Campbell, that's not all dairy can cause. Dr. Campbell attended Cornell on a PhD scholarship, has authored more than 300 research papers, and has *four decades* of high-level research experience. So *The China Study* is, um, a little more intellectual than our book. It's basically the most comprehensive study of diet and nutrition ever conducted in history—spanning twenty years' time; citing from more than 750 references; and partnering Cornell University, Oxford University, and the Chinese Academy of Preventative Medicine! So what does this Holy Grail of nutrition say about dairy? That it can cause heart disease; diabetes; obesity; osteoporosis; kidney stones;

cataracts; macular degeneration; multiple sclerosis; Alzheimer's; and breast, prostate, colon, and rectal cancer![110] Please, read this list again. Slowly. Let each one sink in.

Understandably, you're preoccupied with your pregnancy, and you may not take the time to read *The China Study* right now. Well at some point soon, you really, really should. It's absolutely the most compelling, well-researched, in-depth book on nutrition we've ever come across. In the meantime, we're gonna give you just one of the many pertinent CliffsNotes™ of *The China Study*: Dr. Campbell started a laboratory program to investigate protein's role in the development of cancer. Eventually, due to his diligent, precise, and careful practices, his research received funding for an extraordinary twenty-seven years from the National Institutes of Health, the American Cancer Society, and the American Institute for Cancer Research (among others). In this time, he discovered that protein did indeed have an effect on cancer. "What protein consistently and strongly promoted cancer? Casein, which makes up 87 percent of cows' milk protein, promoted all stages of the cancer process."[111]

There are three stages of cancer he's referring to: initiation, promotion, and progression. Dr. Campbell likens the stages to planting a lawn. "Initiation is when you put the seeds in the soil, promotion is when the grass starts to grow, and progression is when the grass gets completely out of control, invading the driveway, the shrubbery, and the sidewalk." Chemical carcinogens (by-products of industrial processes) are usually what *initiate* normal cells to transform or mutate into cancer-prone cells. *Promotion* is when the cells "multiply until they become a visibly detectable cancer." And *progression* occurs when the cancer cells grow and spread.[112] Let us repeat: Casein, a milk protein, promoted all three stages of cancer growth. Incredibly interesting: His studies showed that exposure to toxic chemicals initiated cancer growth. But the cancer remained dormant and wasn't of issue. However, with the introduction of casein, milk protein, all that changed.[113] Honestly, if you aren't seeing red *now*, you're a lost cause.

Please go back and reread Dr. Campbell's credentials and the background information about *The China Study* once more. Acknowledge that *The China Study* isn't some hole-filled, half-baked, fluff piece, but that it's the real deal. Now get on board. Seriously. This is no joke. This is literally a matter of life and death. Do not dismiss this information just because it seems outlandish and hard to believe. Or just because your doctors and schoolteachers told you otherwise. According to a Senate investigation, doctors receive *less than three hours* of nutritional training in medical school![114] And unsuspecting teachers are puppets whose strings are pulled by the dairy industry. The dairy industry is a for-profit, commercial business, just like Pepsi or McDonald's. Imagine, however, if Pepsi or McDonald's were allowed to provide schools with educational materials regarding nutrition. Unimaginable, right? Because more than likely, soda and Big Macs would be touted as important dietary staples. It'd probably sound a little something like this: "Pepsi has water in it, and it's vital to drink eight glasses of water a day. Big Macs are high in protein, and protein is an important component of any diet." We'd never stand for that, right? But we stand for the dairy industry—a for-profit enterprise—providing lesson plans, educational kits, posters, videos, and teaching guides to thousands of schools![115] And we allow them to sell milk at practically every school in the country! Doctors and teachers aren't dimwits or villains. They're just like the rest of us. It has been so ingrained into each one of us that "Milk does a body good," that no one would ever think to question it.

And because we've all been brainwashed, our children suffer. According to the Physicians Committee for Responsible Medicine (PCRM), "Insulin-dependent diabetes (Type I or childhood-onset) is linked to consumption of dairy products. Epidemiological studies of various countries show a strong correlation between the use of dairy products and the incidence of insulin-dependent diabetes. Researchers in 1992 found that a specific dairy protein sparks an auto-immune reaction, which is believed to be what destroys the insulin-producing cells of the pancreas."[116]

Mammals need the enzyme lactase to digest lactose (the sugar found in dairy). However, between the ages of eighteen months and four years, we lose 90 to 95 percent of this enzyme.[117] So basically, we are *all* lactose-intolerant for the most part. If you took a two-week long hiatus from all dairy, and then reintroduced it, you'd see how shitty it makes you feel. Now imagine your poor child's little body. Hey kid, got colic? If you're feeding your baby cows' milk or you're consuming dairy and breastfeeding, you'll both pay the price. A colicky baby is not happy or fun to be around. Imagine giving your baby a bottle full of giraffe milk and the physical distress it would likely cause her. Why on earth would cows' milk be any different? Just because people have been doing it for years? Or because your doctor said it was okay? Or because you "turned out fine" and you drank it? Get your head out of your ass and use some common sense, please, for the sake of your child. If you do, you'll spend less time at the pediatrician dealing with colic, ear infections, respiratory problems, and skin conditions.[118] And your child won't grow up to be an insolent teenager with acne-prone skin, attention deficit disorder, attention deficit hyperactivity disorder, irritable bowel syndrome, and anxiety, all of which can be attributed to dairy.[119]

If you *keep* your head up your ass, your kid is more likely to suffer from allergies. Milk is the leading cause of allergies in children.[120] Our bodies want nothing to do with dairy. Again, if you took a two-week hiatus from it and then reintroduced it, you'd see just what happens. More than likely, you'd experience a stuffy nose and a ton of mucus, your chest and lungs would feel tight, and your stomach would feel like shit. The more dairy you consume, the more likely you are to see these symptoms. People with dairy allergies who insist on consuming dairy products often develop asthma, as well.[121] Now, again, imagine wreaking all this havoc on the small body of a child . . . and telling her how good it is to drink milk. Be sure to

remind her of this when she's painfully and chronically constipated, too.[122] Or when she has cramping stomachaches, gas,
and diarrhea.[123]

A TALL GLASS OF BOVINE GROWTH HORMONE

Let's pretend for a moment that cows' milk is healthy for
humans. Even if it were—it's not—but even if it were, it
would only be healthy in its purest, unadulterated form. Just
like human breast milk is. But we sure as hell don't consume
cows' milk in its purest, unadulterated form. Nowadays, cows
are injected with bovine growth hormone (BGH). (BGH
milk is also referred to as rBGH—recombinant Bovine
Growth Hormone—or GE—genetically engineered.) Fifty
years ago, the average milk production rate of a cow was
2,000 pounds a year. Today, the top producers provide up to
50,000 pounds a year![124] This is far from natural. (Imagine
being injected with some crazy-ass hormone that would make
your boobs pump out *twenty-five* times more milk than they
would on their own.)

Dr. Samuel Epstein, professor emeritus of Environmental and
Occupational Medicine at the School of Public Health at the
University of Illinois at Chicago, has authored or coauthored

thirteen books, published nearly 300 peer-reviewed scientific articles, and is the leading international expert on BGH. He's also an internationally recognized authority on the mechanisms of carcinogenesis, the causes and prevention of cancer, and the toxic and carcinogenic effects of environmental pollutants. (And he has, like, a million letters after his name: MD, D Path., DTM&H.) Dr. Epstein literally wrote "the book" on BGH: *What's in Your Milk?*[125] The beginning of his BGH journey started with a phone call he received from an angry farmer in 1989. The farmer was involved in the secret testing trials for BGH, and he wanted any scientific information available on the hormone. When Dr. Epstein professed ignorance about the hormone, the farmer responded angrily to the effect of, "If it makes my cows sick, their milk will also make people sick. So it's damn well your job to find out." So Dr. Epstein began his inquiry. Six months later, he received a package that was sent anonymously. Its contents appeared to be records stolen directly from the FDA files—confidential data from BGH trials. And they included information that had been previously undisclosed, revealing a wide range of serious veterinary dangers associated with BGH.[126] You shouldn't be surprised to learn that the shit surrounding BGH is every bit as shady as aspartame's. Especially because Monsanto, the same company that owned NutraSweet, is the giant behind BGH. (BGH is sold to farmers under the trade name POSILAC.)[127] Dr. Epstein sent copies of the incriminating documents to Congressman John Conyers, who publicly stated, "Monsanto and the FDA have chosen to suppress and manipulate animal health test data . . . in efforts to approve commercial use of rBGH."[128]

Both Monsanto and the FDA knowingly and falsely claimed that:

1. There is no difference between milk from BGH cows and untreated cows.

Um, bullshit. According to Dr. Epstein, "GE milk is entirely different from natural milk: nutritionally, biochemically, pharmacologically, and immunologically."[129]

2. BGH is harmless to cows.[130]

Um, bullshit again. Its own package insert lists sixteen harmful health effects![131] And studies showed that cows treated with BGH had chronic inflammation of internal organs, ulcerating injection site reactions, and deep carcass damage. Almost half the injected cows became infertile! And the majority suffered from anemia and chronic mastitis—a bacterial infection resulting from inflamed udders. So what does all this mean? Cows injected with BGH are also treated with antibiotics and other drugs, many unapproved and illegal. During a single lactation period, one cow received 120 drug treatments![132] All lactating mammals excrete toxins through their milk, including hormones, antibiotics, pesticides, and chemicals.[133] So when you consume dairy products from cows treated with BGH, you're ingesting all that shit, too! By the way, approximately *70 percent* of all the antibiotics made in the United States each year are administered to farm animals, causing antibiotic resistance in humans.[134]

3. BGH milk is safe for human consumption.

Triple dose of bullshit! BGH milk has high levels of Insulin Growth Factor (IGF-1), which has been consistently linked to breast, colon, and prostate cancers.[135]

If you weren't pregnant, we'd expect you to be so worked up right now that you'd be spitting blood. We're all being killed slowly so people can shove a fistful of green fucking paper in their greedy-ass pockets.

P.S. A study revealed that women who consumed meat and/or dairy products were *five times* more likely to conceive twins compared with vegan women. Five times! In a recent issue of the *Journal of Reproductive Medicine*, Dr. Gary Steinman, who conducted the study, argued that IGF-1 might be the reason. IGF-1 is a protein that gets released by the liver in response to BGH. Studies show that the protein increases ovulation.[136] S-c-a-r-y.

BGH milk is banned in Australia, New Zealand,[137] all of the European Union, Canada, Japan, and every other industrialized country in the world. Both the World Trade Organization and The United Nations Food Standards Body refuse to endorse the hormone's safety.[138] But BGH is legal in the United States. It's so baffling that we're supposed to be one of the most advanced nations in the world.

PUS, CHEMICALS, OR BOTH?

Got pus? On factory farms, where the majority of our milk comes from, there is no gentle farmer milking cows with a bucket between his feet. Clamps are attached to cows' udders and cows are milked by machine. (Imagine that after having just given birth!) The udders become sore and infected. Pus forms. But the machines keep on milking, sucking the dead white blood cells into the milk. In the good ol' U.S. of A., we have the highest allowable upper limit of pus concentration in the world—almost double the international standard.[139] Instead of saying, "It's as American as apple pie," we can start saying, "It's as American as pus in your milk!" Yeehaw!

Oh yeah, we're not done yet. To get rid of all the pus, bacteria, and other grossness, milk has to be pasteurized. (Meaning, they gotta boil the hell out of it.) So even if cows' milk was good for humans—it isn't—this process destroys beneficial enzymes, makes calcium less available, and creates radioactive particles.[140]

Pus and radioactive particles aren't the only dangers lurking in your milk. Oh no, batting third is dioxin, a known human carcinogen that can negatively impact hormones in fetal development.[141] Dioxins are unintentional by-products from industrial practices (like chemical manufacturing, metal refining, combustion, etc.). They get released into the air and then settle into water (affecting the fish) and onto grasslands (affecting the cattle that graze there). Dioxin gets absorbed into the flesh of the animals exposed to it. So when we eat the animals' flesh or consume the milk of the animals, we get exposed to dioxin. It crosses the placenta during pregnancy and endangers the fetus.[142]

PCBs are other sinister chemicals that accumulate in fat. Like dioxins, PCBs are exceptionally dangerous for developing brains in fetuses and children. Prenatal exposure can have permanent effects on IQ. Dutch researchers even found a link between these pollutants and gender-swapping behaviors. High dietary exposures to PCB had girls displaying "masculine" behaviors and boys displaying "feminine" behaviors. Even though PCBs have been banned in the United States for more than twenty years, they still persist in our environment and will continue to contaminate our meat and dairy for many years.[143]

We're still going. Brominated flame retardants (BFRs) resemble PCBs chemically. Research suggests that BFRs have adverse affects on the brain, liver, and reproductive system, and on thyroid function. Where do these BFR bad boys accumulate? Animal-based foods.[144] A more specific class of BFRs is polybrominated diphenyl ethers (PBDEs). Studies showed PBDEs levels in mothers to be the same as the levels in their cord blood. Meaning, their newborns had the same levels as they did! Researchers believe that prenatal exposure to the chemicals may cause memory, behavior, and learning disorders. It's suggested that PBDE exposure in the United States is among the highest in the world. Flame retardants used in household items pollute our environment. Farm animals and fish absorb these pollutants. When we eat their flesh or drink their milk, we're exposed.[145]

How cute. You want to know why the government and U.S. Department of Agriculture don't protect us from all this? Why would they bother with industrial pollutants when they don't even bat an eye at the pesticides used in raising farm animals or in growing their feed? Sickeningly high levels of pesticides found in dairy meet government standards. Records from the Food and Drug Administration show that "virtually 100 percent of the cheese products produced and sold in the United States has detectable pesticide residues."[146]

DIRTY SECRETS, LEUKEMIA,
AND A WHOLE LOT OF DRAMA

The U.S. government sure as hell doesn't bother with Johne's disease. Oh, wait, you've never heard of it? Of course you haven't. Because Johne's (pronounced Yo Neez) disease is "something that farmers talk about secretly—whisper behind hands." One dairy scientist calls it the "whispering campaign" and stated he had never heard a frank, open discussion about it. One dairy farmer referred to Johne's as "a dirty word. It's like AIDS—you don't talk about it."[147] When the USDA released a report on 2,500 dairy producers in 1997, they estimated that up to 40 percent of those dairy herds were infected. (They also conceded that it was likely an *underestimate*.)[147] Health experts correlate the high rate of Johne's disease in cattle with the growing epidemic of Crohn's disease in humans.[147] How is it transmitted? People suffering from Crohn's disease suffer from uncontrollable diarrhea. And apparently, cows with Johne's disease suffer the same affliction. (Get your barf bag handy.) The diarrhea can come shooting out of the cow in liquid form. And because her butt is so close to her udders, poo gets on her udders. And unless someone takes the time to wash and clean the udders of every cow before every milking, the infected fecal matter makes its way into the milk. Bonus: Within that poo, there can be as many as one trillion para-tuberculosis bugs per gram. Surprise, surprise: The good ol' U.S. of A. has the highest incidence of Crohn's disease in the world.[147] Hey, instead of, "It's as American as pus in your milk," it can be, "It's as American as poopy milk and Crohn's disease."

Unless we want to change it to, "It's as American as leukemia." The bovine leukemia virus involves about 80 percent of dairy herds! The virus can be killed if the milk is pasteurized, and pasteurized correctly. But sometimes milk is sold "raw." In a study of randomly collected raw samples, the virus was detected in *two thirds*![148] Now you're probably thinking, "Oh, phew. I don't buy raw milk products." But what if the milk you do buy isn't pasteurized correctly? Or what if the milk processing plant has an accidental "cross contamination" between raw and pasteurized milk? Unfortunately, states with known leukemic dairy herds have higher rates of human leukemia.[149]

It's all too unbelievable, right? We know. But bear in mind we have nothing to gain by telling you all this. In fact, we've got everything to lose. The billion-dollar dairy industry is so rich and powerful, they could sue us for everything we have.

(Remember when the cattle ranchers sued Oprah, unsuccessfully, for publicly disparaging beef?) It would cost them next to nothing, but the legal fees would bankrupt us in minutes. We're risking our own livelihoods to tell you this. So don't be skeptical of us, like we're trying to sell you the Brooklyn Bridge. You've already bought the book, so whether you believe us or not doesn't add any money to our coffers. We're telling you this and hoping you'll believe it, because it's true. And because we can't bear that *anyone* would eat and drink this poison, let alone pregnant women!

By the way, don't think you can worm your way out of the dairy drama by eating "low-fat" dairy products. They're still made from cows' milk, so they're just as pus-y, grody, and contaminated. Not to mention they can affect your friggin' fertility! A new study of 18,555 women found that those who ate two or more servings of low-fat dairy products a day had almost *double* the risk of infertility.[150] Frightening. In addition, low-fat and fat-free dairy products can have a relative overburden of protein and lactose. Too much protein can tax the kidneys and leach calcium from the bones.[151] And undigested lactose encourages the growth of bacteria in our intestines.[152] Gross.

ORGANIC DAIRY SUCKS

Sorry, dairy queens, but organic dairy products aren't much better. You've let the dairy industry dupe you long enough. Don't dupe yourself! Don't allow your addiction to cheese or your outdated beliefs con you into thinking that organic dairy is some clean, pure, magical entity. These products *may* be free of the chemical pesticides, hormones, and antibiotics, but they too can have fecal matter and pus. And in case you forgot everything you just read in this chapter: The consumption of dairy has been linked to heart disease; diabetes; obesity; osteoporosis; kidney stones; cataracts; macular degeneration; multiple sclerosis; Alzheimer's; and breast, prostate, colon, and rectal cancer![153] Use your head! Cows' milk is for baby cows; it is not good for humans! (Even if it was, how would you like it if right after you give birth someone snatched your baby away, attached clamps to your nipples, milked you, and then sold your milk for profit? The fact that they are "just" cows doesn't make it any less cruel or sadistic.)

UM, WHAT'S THE POINT OF MILK, AGAIN?

Okay, so you know you don't need milk for calcium, but what

about vitamin D? Well, milk can't be trusted for that, either! According to PCRM, "Samplings of milk have found a significant variation of vitamin D content, with some samplings having had as much as 500 times the indicated level, while others had little or none at all." FYI: Too much vitamin D can be toxic![154] But it's been reported that "vitamin D is routinely added to milk 'above and beyond' the legal requirements."[155] Don't get us wrong—vitamin D is important, especially for pregnant women. It aids in calcium and phosphorous absorption. But you don't need to play Russian roulette with cows' milk to get it. Just get off your ass, open your door, and go outside. The body makes vitamin D when the skin is exposed to the sun! How cool is that? (Depending on your skin tone and locale, you just need five to twenty minutes of sun a day, two to seven days a week on your face and hands.)[156] However, be advised that many pregnant women (and people in general) don't get enough sunlight due to their lifestyles. And that sunscreen that protects against skin cancer also blocks the rays needed to make vitamin D. So be sure to eat vitamin D-fortified foods, like cereals, rice-, and soy milks, or talk to your doctor about a vegan vitamin D supplement. (After you find out what you need, visit vegetarian vitamin.com or veganessentials.com.)

How 'bout those minerals? Fruits and veggies have higher levels of iron, manganese, selenium, and chromium than milk. And again, they're more absorbable from these sources than from milk.[157] Just eat a variety of colorful fruits and veggies and snack on raw nuts and seeds every day. And feel great about it. Each bite is a gift to yourself and your baby!

Calcium is naturally abundant in and most readily absorbed from leafy greens (kale, mustard greens, collard greens, turnip greens), bok choy, cabbage, broccoli, Brussels sprouts, okra, watercress, chickpeas, red beans, soybeans, almonds, sesame seeds, and sea vegetables (like seaweed). It can also be attained from fortified orange juice, soymilk, rice milk, cereal, and calcium-processed tofu. And these foods don't come laden with fat, cholesterol, and a harmful excess of protein. These foods are nothing but good for ya.

Pregnant women should aim for 1,000 milligrams of calcium per day.[158] But don't think you can eat crap all day and then just pop a calcium supplement to make up for it. There's no substitute for healthy, calcium-rich foods. So take your viteys, if instructed, but eat well, too. Have four servings per day of calcium-rich foods.[159]

How do you know if you're not getting enough calcium? Nighttime leg cramps may indicate an imbalance of calcium, magnesium, phosphorous,[160] or iron.[161] Other symptoms can include heart palpitations, insomnia, depression, nerve sensitivity, twitching, brittle nails, and numbness in the fingers or toes.[162] There are cases where people don't experience these symptoms, but still have a calcium deficiency. However, provided you're healthy and not on any "calcium-wasting" meds, and if you're meeting your calorie needs with whole plant foods (fresh fruits, veggies, leafy greens, nuts, seeds, whole-grains, and legumes), you should be fine.

Now, if you're anything like us, eating gives you more joy than anything—even making babies. So you might be wondering, "What the hell am I gonna eat now that I know dairy is bad for me and my baby? I know how to get calcium, but how about pleasure?" Don't worry. We're on it! First off, soymilk, rice milk, and almond milk are great replacements for cows' milk. Just read the ingredients and make sure the one you buy is fortified or enriched (that means they added calcium and other good stuff). Also, avoid brands that have any form of sweeteners in the "milk." If you're trying to limit your sugar intake, you sure as hell don't want to waste your ration on friggin' rice milk—you want naughty food. Next, get yourself some soy butter. It tastes like the real deal and can be used just like butter—on toast, in mashed potatoes, even in recipes. Mmm! We could eat it with a spoon! Speaking of . . . Have you tried soy ice cream? Seriously, it'll rock your world. Yes, you should be limiting your sugar intake, but if you *have* to have ice cream, rock the soy. It is ridiculously good. Tofutti makes pretty decent dairy-free versions of cream cheese and sour cream. And the best dairy-free cheese on the market is Follow Your Heart. Feel free to try other brands, but read the ingredients. The majority of soy cheeses on the market *aren't* dairy-free. Some contain casein, which is the milk protein that promotes all three stages of cancer growth, remember? Others contain whey. Uck. But Follow Your Heart receives our stamp of approval. If you can't find good stuff at your local store, venture out to the nearest health food store or Whole Foods. Or, flap your big gums and ask your store's manager to order the stuff for you. They'll usually accommodate special requests. (Especially if you rub your pregnant belly while you ask.) If you're like most people, you've been buying the same crappy products for years. So be patient: It'll take a little time to locate all the dairy-free products, and it'll require trial and error to figure out which ones you like.

So yeah, we just told you that dairy products suck for you and your baby. Don't freak out. Going against the grain can feel uncomfortable, wrong, and downright frightening. After all, every doctor you've ever known has endorsed milk's safety and nutritional value. Unfortunately, they simply don't know any better. But bear in mind, there are many, many, many health experts, scientists, researchers, and doctors who vehemently oppose the claims of the dairy industry. Their voices are just drowned out by the billion-dollar industry. If what we've said in this chapter kinda rings true for you, but you still feel uncomfortable, do your own research. Take matters into your own hands. Collecting information can be the ultimate reassurance. It's disquieting to believe what others say, but when you've seen the proof yourself, it's a whole new ballgame.

To help get the ball rolling, we'll leave you with this: Dr. John McDougall is a physician and nutrition expert with more than thirty years of experience. He's also the founder and medical director of the nationally renowned McDougall Program, and the author of several national bestsellers, including *The McDougall Program for Women*. He says, "When a pregnant American woman thinks about adding calcium to her body, she automatically thinks she needs to drink more milk. Yet after they are weaned from their mothers, billions of women worldwide consume no milk and produce perfectly healthy and strong children." [163]

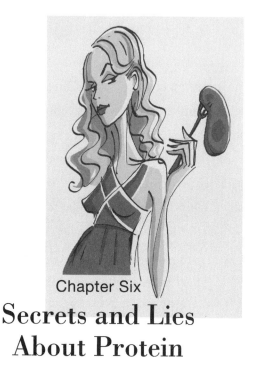

Chapter Six

Secrets and Lies About Protein

With all the low-carb bullshit going on in this country, it's never been more necessary to establish the facts about protein. First and foremost, everyone seems to think that protein exists just to help build muscle—like protein is the big muscle-head at the gym. Yes, protein does form muscle tissue, but it also has many more functions than that. Protein assures proper growth, maintenance, and repair of *all* body tissues (not just muscles). It also contributes to healing the body; production of blood cells, energy, and hormones; the formation of antibodies and hemoglobin; and the building of enzymes.[164] Those who don't get enough protein can suffer from decreased immunity, loss of muscle mass, improper growth, and weakening of the heart and respiratory system.[165]

So clearly, protein is an important part of any diet. But it shouldn't be the cornerstone of any diet, and this is where the high-protein/low-carb craze really misleads people. You know by now that complex carbs shouldn't be forsaken. But should you overload on protein? Hell, no. Did you have trouble getting pregnant? Studies have shown that excessive protein—especially animal protein—can cause elevated levels of ammonium in the reproductive tract.[166] Harvard researchers studied fertility in more than 18,000 women and found that "Ovulation infertility was 39 percent more likely in women with the highest intake of animal protein than in those with the lowest. The reverse was true for women with the highest intake of plant protein, who were substantially less likely to have had ovulatory infertility than women with the lowest plant protein intake."[167] And according to a recent study published in the *International Journal of Cancer*, animal fat and protein increase the risk of endometrial cancer.[168] Jacked-up levels of protein aren't good for anyone—especially pregnant women and developing babies. It was reported in *The Journal of Endocrinology & Metabolism* that a maternal high-protein/low-carb diet can have adverse effects on the fetus, reduce birth weight, and cause higher adult blood pressures for the offspring later in life.[169] A study presented at the European Congress of Endocrinology revealed more bad news for protein junkies. In the late 1960s, a group of pregnant women were advised to eat high-protein/low-carb diets. It was discovered that the more meat they ate late in the pregnancy, the higher the cortisol levels were in their now-adult offspring. Cortisol is a stress hormone! And in addition to causing stress, high cortisol levels can lead to diabetes.[170] Happy birthday! Mommy loves you so much, she got you high blood pressure, stress, *and* diabetes!

Not even taking Atkins dieters into account, Americans eat about *double* the amount of protein needed. So how many grams of protein do non-pregnant humans need each day? Use this simple equation to find out:

Body weight (in pounds) x .36= recommended protein intake.[171]

While pregnant (or breastfeeding), you should aim for an

additional ten grams of protein a day. But they sure as hell shouldn't come from deli/luncheon/smoked/cured/processed meats like bacon, ham, hot dogs, bologna, salami, etc. (Or smoked fish!) These can contain nitrates or nitrites (food additives), which can cause childhood leukemia[172] or brain tumors.[173]

And they definitely shouldn't come from eggs, either! An Argentine study found that people who ate about one and a half eggs per week had almost *five* times the risk of colorectal cancer as those who ate less than eleven eggs a year. After analyzing data from thirty-four different countries, the World Health Organization correlated egg consumption with death from colon and rectal cancers. Another study found that moderate egg consumption *tripled* the risk of developing bladder cancer. And several studies have associated (incidence of and mortality from) ovarian cancer with egg consumption![174] So save your, "But what about organic, free-range eggs?" bullshit for someone else—someone who doesn't care about your colon, rectum, bladder, and ovaries.

So where *should* this protein come from? Like any average American, your brain probably went back to the muscle-head at the gym, and you likely thought, "I need to get X grams of

protein a day. I'll just eat more chicken, meat, or fish."
(Notice we left dairy off that list. If you still want to consume
dairy products after that last chapter, we're gonna kick your
fat ass.) Somehow, we've all been conditioned into thinking
(dairy), chicken, meat, and fish are the only foods in existence
that have protein. However, this is simply not the case. And
it's a good thing. Because these foods present multiple health
risks to you and your developing fetus.

JUST. PLAIN. GROSS.

For starters, according to the USDA, 70 percent of all food
poisoning is caused by contaminated animal flesh.[175] There
are all sorts of gross things you can get from eating meat,
chicken, eggs, and fish (or from foods that touch these foods).
You may've heard of toxoplasmosis, the disease you can get
from changing your kitty's litter box. But did you know you
could also get it from eating raw or undercooked meat? It's
caused by a microscopic parasite that's not only gross, but also
dangerous to your unborn baby. Toxoplasmosis can cause
miscarriage, stillbirth, loss of vision, loss of hearing, mental
retardation, and death.[176] Listeria is no laughing matter,
either. It can be found in raw meat, eggs, and dairy products;

minimally processed cheeses (like feta, brie, and roquefort); pâtés; and foods that have come into contact with these foods.[177] It too can cause miscarriage, stillbirth, or premature birth.[178] You've all heard of salmonella, but how about campylobacter? Well, Consumer Reports tested store-bought broiler chickens nationwide and found salmonella and/or campylobacter contamination in nearly *half* of them, including those from organic, free-range, and kosher producers![179] You can also get salmonella from raw or undercooked eggs or products containing them. If you do get salmonella, be on the lookout for diarrhea, arthritis, colon damage, and the Grim Reaper.[180] E. coli is no picnic, either, and can be caught by ingesting raw dairy products or improperly cooked meat. Just so you know, the presence of E. Coli is an indicator of fecal contamination. How'd you like a side of shit with those fries? A USDA study found detectable levels of E. Coli in more than 99 percent of store-bought broiler chickens![181] Once infected, a person can expect bloody diarrhea and possibly even renal failure.[182] Oh, but don't worry. Processors spray chicken carcasses with disinfectant—inside and out.[183] (Gag! How'd you like a can of Lysol with those wings?)

SEX, DRUGS, AND FACTORY FARMS

Well, even if we do get food poisoning, we can just take medicine, right? Hmm. Of the *ten billion* animals slaughtered each year in America, the vast majority comes from factory farms. Factory farms that raise cattle, pigs, chickens, egg-laying hens, veal calves, or dairy cows keep an enormous amount of animals in a very small space. There are few vast meadows or lush, green pastures. The animals are confined inside buildings, where they are literally packed in on top of each other. Egg-laying hens are crammed into cages so small, they can barely open their wings, and their feet get mangled from the wire mesh floors. Pigs and cows are kept in stalls so small, they are unable to turn around or lie down comfortably. Broiler chickens are crowded so tightly into warehouse-type structures that they often peck each other to death. Animals live in the filth of their own urine, feces, and vomit with infected, festering sores and wounds. To keep them alive in these unsanitary conditions, factory farmers give animals regular doses of antibiotics.[184] But they don't sort through ten billion animals to see who's sick and might need it. They give it to all of them. Penicillin, tetracycline, and countless other antibiotics are routinely administered. When we eat the flesh of these animals, we're eating these antibiotics. Approximately *70 percent* of all the antibiotics used in the United States each year is given to farm animals![185]

This overuse of antibiotics leads to the development of new antibiotic-resistant bacterial strains. Meaning, due to the abuse of antibiotics by factory farmers, new bacterial strains are forming (gross) and the antibiotics we'd normally take to combat them are rendered ineffective (scary). One USDA study found 67 percent of chicken and 66 percent of beef to be contaminated with "superbugs" that couldn't be killed by antibiotics.[186] Nasty. No wonder the European Union wants nothing to do with our meat. They only allow four antibiotics to be used on their livestock, none of which are used in human health care. Does Lady Liberty have any restrictions like these? Nope.[187] Our country allows farmers to feed arsenic to broiler chickens. You heard us. It's legal to *feed arsenic* to broiler chickens (to kill parasites and promote growth). Apparently, the USDA and FDA don't mind that researchers found arsenic residue in chicken at 100 percent of fast-food restaurants and 50 percent of supermarkets investigated.[188] Gnarly.

On factory farms, animals are raised in the smallest quarters possible, where they're "grown" as large as possible to inflate the profit margin as much as possible. In addition to antibiotics and arsenic, anabolic steroids are routinely administered to the animals. It's been reported that approximately 99 percent of commercially raised cattle is treated with growth hormones![189] When we eat their flesh, we're eating the growth hormones. No wonder Americans are struggling with weight problems—we're ingesting growth hormones on a regular basis.

And no wonder reproductive cancers have skyrocketed since the 1950s—breast cancer has increased by 55 percent, testicular cancer has gone up by 120 percent, and prostate cancer has increased 190 percent![190] In addition to antibiotics and steroids, growth-promoting sex hormones are also given to farm animals routinely. For more than a decade, the FDA has allowed farmers to implant hormonal agents in the ears of cows. These include—but are in no way limited to—testosterone (male hormone); estradiol and progesterone (female hormones); and norgestomet (a synthetic progestin).[191] By the way, the estrogen estradiol is one of the most commonly used hormones for fattening cows. And it's a potent carcinogen.[192] S-c-a-r-y. Even scarier: A USDA survey of feedlots found that nearly half the cows had illegally misplaced implants in their muscle tissue, as opposed to their ears. (Let us add that the statistic represents the implants that were *visibly* misplaced.[193] The actual percentage could've been well above half.) These hormones can contribute to estrogen dominance, which has been linked to endometriosis; fibroids; and breast, ovarian, and cervical cancer in women. In men, estrogen dominance can cause prostate and testicular cancer, and even "male menopause." Don't laugh. Male menopause can include symptoms like impotence, testicular atrophy, breast growth, fatigue, depression, and reduction or loss of sex drive. Who's at the highest risk for male menopause? Those who worked on poultry farms, implanting chickens and turkeys with estrogen pellets![194] You do the math.

In Puerto Rico in the early 1980s, after eating meat from treated cows, thousands of children developed painful ovarian cysts and experienced premature sexual growth.[195] A new study in *Human Reproduction* reported that the more meat women ate while pregnant, the lower their sons' sperm concentration![196] And nowadays, 15 percent of Caucasian and nearly 50 percent of African American girls start puberty at the age of eight![197]

It just keeps getting worse. The Pentagon commissioned

a series of tests on Zeranol, one of the most commonly implanted synthetic estrogens. Researchers reported "significant" cancer cell growth and questioned a link between Zeranol and breast cancer. The European Union bans hormones in beef.[198] The United States? Bon appétit!

MAD COW DISEASE, CHEMICALS. . . WHEN DOES IT END?

Unfortunately, that's not the only area the United States is lacking in regarding meat safety issues. In Japan, 100 percent of cattle slaughtered for human consumption are tested for mad cow disease.[199] Here, we test approximately .0010428 percent.[200] (For those of you who are mathematically challenged, that's less than one-tenth of one percent!) Former Agriculture Secretary Mike Johanns admitted that testing is not done to protect consumers from mad cow disease, but rather to discern the disease's prevalence.[201] How reassuring. Hmm, we wonder if that's why 65 nations have full or partial restrictions on importing our beef.[202] It could be that. Or it could be that the FDA approved the spraying of live viruses onto meat and poultry products (to combat listeria). Yeah, the spray contains six different viral strains and meat companies aren't obligated to inform customers which products have been sprayed.[203]

Unfortunately, even if the USDA and FDA implemented bans on hormones, steroids, and antibiotics, our meat would still be contaminated with toxic chemicals. Here's how it works—Pesticides 101: Pesticides are used on crops to prevent bugs from destroying them. If it's a crop grown for us to eat, we wash them off, getting rid of some of the chemicals. If it's a crop used to feed animals, the pesticides are not washed off. And unlike crops grown for us to eat, crops grown for animals to eat have no limits on the amount of pesticides that can be used. More than one billion pounds of pesticides are used each year in this country![204] And approximately 80 percent are used on the four major animal-feed crops.[205] P.S. Pesticides are also sprayed directly onto the animals themselves to ward off parasites, insects, rodents, and fungi. So, you can see, the animals we're ingesting are subject to major pesticide ingestion and exposure for their entire lives. And when we ingest the animals, we're ingesting the pesticides, too. What you can't see is that the animals store these pesticides in their fat tissue and cells.[206] So when you eat meat, you're ingesting a higher amount of pesticides than you would if you ate the pesticide-treated food directly.

And unfortunately, pesticides aren't all we're getting. Herbicides, industrial wastes, PCBs, BFRs, BDFEs—they're polluting our waterways and affecting our food supply. But again, the fatty tissues of animals attract and concentrate these chemicals—"bio-accumulation." And as all these environmental pollutants move up the food chain, they're concentrated even more—"biomagnification."[207] So a corn crop may have a specific amount of toxic residue in it. Then a cow, chicken, or pig eats the corn and absorbs a larger amount of toxic residue. Then a human eats the cow, chicken, or pig and absorbs an even larger amount of toxic residue.

Just one of these chemicals on its own would be scary enough. But the abundance and complex interaction of so many can wreak havoc on our endocrine, hormonal, neurological, immunological, and reproductive systems.[208] Imagine what these toxins can do to developing fetuses. Prenatal exposure has caused altered sexual behavior, like demasculinization and feminization; behavioral problems; learning disabilities; hyperactivity; under-activity; memory problems; growth retardation; delayed reflexes; reduced intelligence;[209] limb deformities; heart defects; penis deformities; undescended testicles; reduced size of penis and testicles; eye inflammation; and hyperpigmentation.[210] Infants and children are also at a much higher risk than adults because their organs are still growing and developing, and they eat and drink more than adults in relation to their body weights (so their exposure to toxins can be higher, relatively speaking).[211] Destruction, disruptions, and alterations during these delicate developmental periods can cause permanent and irreversible damage, especially because their metabolic pathways and immune systems are immature. There is an increased risk for childhood cancers and for neurological diseases later in life, like dementia and Parkinson's.[212]

SOMETHING'S FISHY

Sadly, our waters aren't any better; they too are alarmingly polluted. So eating fish (or other seafood) is just as dangerous as eating meat. Their flesh also accumulates and absorbs chemical pollutants, like mercury, organochlorides, PCBs, and others. It works like this: Chemical levels in water may be low enough to receive passing grades from the Environmental Protection Agency (EPA). But the chemical concentration in algae can increase by up to 250. When the zooplankton eats the algae, the concentration can double. When the tiny shrimp eat the zooplankton, the concentration can be 45,000 times higher. By the time the little fish eat the shrimp, and the big fish eat the little fish, and we eat the big fish, we're looking at a concentration 25 million times that which was found in the water![213]

For so long, fish was seen as the "golden child" of the protein world. But in 2001 and again in 2004, when the FDA and EPA issued a fish advisory for kids; pregnant women; breast-feeding moms; and women planning to get pregnant, a brief shadow was cast on seafood. At the time, it was suggested that these groups should severely limit their intake of canned tuna and completely avoid fish like swordfish and mackerel. But some scientists felt that the advisory was too lenient and that it was more in favor of industry relations than consumer safety. One university toxicology expert resigned from the FDA advisory panel, claiming, "The new recommendations are dangerous to 99 percent of pregnant women and their unborn children. It seems that one should be more concerned about the health of the future children of this country than the albacore tuna industry." One in six women in the United States have enough mercury in their blood to put their babies at risk. Mercury can deform fetuses, reduce IQ and motor skills, and cause damage to the central nervous system. Studies revealed that mothers who consumed high amounts of fish had children that were slower to walk and talk.[214] Yet, in October 2007, despite all the damning evidence against fish, the National Healthy Mothers, Healthy Babies Coalition issued an advisory recommending pregnant women eat *at least* twelve ounces of fish and seafood per week. (The EPA/FDA advised *no more than* twelve ounces per week.) Their concern was that pregnant moms and developing fetuses need omega-3 acids and DHA, which we agree with.[215] However, there are other sources for both (which we delve into in the Stupid, Boring Vitamin chapter) that don't come laden with mercury and other toxins. But because the report was commissioned by the seafood industry and funded by $74,000 from the National Fisheries Institute,[216] we wouldn't expect them to discuss those alternatives. Hell, some of the group's "members" (like the American Academy of Pediatrics, the Centers for Disease Control and Prevention, and the March of Dimes) didn't even know the report existed until it was published, after which they opposed its recommendations.[217] But hey, screw it, your doctor will probably tell you to avoid sushi, but that six ounces per week of canned tuna is fine. And she'll be wearing a white lab coat and stethoscope. So just disregard the fact that high mercury levels in fish-eating moms have been linked with birth defects, seizures, mental retardation, developmental disabilities, and cerebral palsy.[218] Don't bother doing your own research and looking into the issue yourself.

And if you really feel like kidding yourself, pretend "farm-raised" fish are clean and pure. Cover your ears when we say that the feed given to farm-raised salmon has high levels of chemical pollutants, making them practically toxic in comparison to ocean-caught fish (which you now know are polluted).[219] Close your eyes to the fact that the farmed salmon are fed artificial dyes to make them appear pink like wild salmon, instead of the unnatural, murky gray color they actually are.[220]

Tell yourself that "everything in moderation" is fine, and that some fish contain beneficial omega-3 fatty acids. Hell, everyone says you should eat fish two or three times a week for heart-healthy omega-3s, right? Um, actually, no, not everyone. A recent study in the *British Medical Journal* reported that eating fish did *not* have a beneficial effect on heart health.[221] Perhaps that's because some fish can be high in cholesterol and saturated fat. Disregard that you can get omega-3s from eating walnuts, which have no cholesterol and are low in saturated fat. And by all means, pay no mind to the *American Journal of Cardiology* study that praised walnuts' positive effect on arteries.[222]

FRIGGIN' PROTEIN

Whether it's milk, cheese, eggs, chicken, pork, beef, or fish, animal foods are the only ones that have cholesterol. They also contain fat and saturated fat. And that's in addition to all the bacteria, hormones, steroids, pesticides, chemical pollutants, and antibiotics! Um, so why do we eat them—for protein? Yep, basically, we risk heart disease, obesity, diabetes, all sorts of cancers, and the health of our unborn babies because we've been brainwashed into thinking these are the only foods with protein. But we can easily obtain adequate protein by eating a variety of fruits, vegetables, whole grains, nuts, seeds, and legumes. And it just so happens that those foods have a variety of health benefits, too! For you and baby! Eat all types of beans, peas, lentils, nuts, and seeds; breads and pastas made from whole grains; bulgur; millet; barley; quinoa; buckwheat; oats; amaranth; brown rice; potatoes;

sweet potatoes; broccoli; kale; asparagus; avocados; soybeans; tofu—the list is endless, really. Fruits. Veggies.
Legumes. Nuts. Seeds. Whole grains. All sources of protein.

And contrary to popular belief (surprise, surprise), meat is
not the only "complete" protein. Meaning, soybeans also
have all the amino acids our bodies can't produce on their
own.[223] But even if you don't eat soy, you can get all the
aminos by eating a variety of fruits, veggies, legumes, nuts,
seeds, and whole grains. And it doesn't have to be in one sitting. As long as you're eating a variety of foods from those
food groups, you're getting all the aminos you need![224] So pick
something else to be neurotic about.

THE SOY SAGA

Should you eat soy or shouldn't you? There's so much controversy surrounding soy, it's hard to know what to believe and
what the real "truth" is. Supporters claim it can do everything—lower cholesterol, reduce heart disease, and decrease
risk of multiple cancers. Opponents claim it can depress thyroid function, block mineral absorption, and cause cancer.[225]
Here's what we know to be "pro-soy true":

• Soybeans are "complete proteins," meaning they contain

the essential amino acids our bodies don't manufacture.[226]

- Calorie for calorie, soybeans have twice as much protein as red meat and cheese, and ten times more protein than whole milk.[227]

- Soybeans are a good source of omega-3 fatty acids.[228]

- Soybeans have more iron, calcium, phosphorous, and B vitamins than eggs.[229]

- The majority of studies claiming soy has negative effects were conducted on animals. And animal tests are simply unreliable indicators, as the biology of each species varies greatly. (Cases in point: Thalidomide tested safe in animals, but caused horrendous birth defects in children. Diet phenom "fen fen" tested safe in animals, but caused heart abnormalities in humans. Arthritis drug Opren tested safe in animals but killed humans!)[230]

- Entire civilizations have been eating soy for thousands of years without any ill effects and, in fact, have lower instances of cancer and heart disease.

Here's what we know to be "anti-soy true":

- None of these civilizations have been eating as much soy as we eat now.

- None of these civilizations have been eating soy in so many highly processed forms. They've been eating tofu, tempeh, miso, and actual soybeans. Here and now, we have soy "meats," "cheeses," "ice creams," and even supplements. And soybean oil makes its way into a multitude of processed foods.
- Soy is one of the most common genetically engineered crops around. So unless you're buying organic, you're probably eating soybeans that have been genetically manipulated.
- Soy is one of the highest pesticide-laden crops around. So unless you're buying organic, you're getting a hefty dose of pesticides.

So what's all the drama about? Basically, it centers on isoflavones and phytoestrogens, chemical compounds found in soybeans (and other plant foods, too). Because isoflavones and phytoestrogens structurally resemble human estrogens, and estrogen can have an effect on breast tissue, their safety has been questioned. According to soy supporters, however, anti-soy studies use an isolated, concentrated amount of soy isoflavones that exceed what a person would consume. And again, the studies showing negative effects are conducted on animals, who metabolize soy differently than we do. (Case in point: Humans can eat chocolate without incidence. However, chocolate can be fatal when ingested by dogs.)[231] In addition, when you extract certain components of many foods and test them in isolation, they can be harmful. But when eaten as part of whole foods in normal-sized servings, they are perfectly safe. Mushrooms, broccoli, lentils, grapefruits, peanuts, spinach, chard, and celery are all examples of this. Broccoli, lentils, and grapefruit have naturally occurring pesticides, which, if you extracted and ate in their concentrated forms in high doses, can cause mutations. Mushrooms contain carcinogens. Peanuts can harbor traces of aflatoxin, cancer-causing substances. Spinach and chard contain an acid that can diminish calcium absorption. And celery has toxins that can damage the immune system.[232] But these are all healthy foods. And the sums of all their parts offer protection from the potential dangers of one or two individual components. It's when we start tinkering with their chemistry that we see "dangers." So it isn't surprising to see breast cancer cells in mice who are dosed with a thousand milligrams of soy isoflavones.

Another common accusation is that soy has a negative

impact on thyroid function. However, only one adult human study conducted in Japan over fifteen years ago has concluded that. (And better-designed and more recent studies done in the United States did not support those findings.)[233] Every day for three months straight, seventeen people were fed thirty grams of pickled, roasted soybeans. Half of these participants experienced either an enlargement of the thyroid *or* a hypothyroidism symptom, like fatigue or constipation.[234] Does eight or nine people (some experiencing only fatigue or constipation) prove that soy has a negative effect on thyroid function?

So, a lot of the negative hype around soy is bullshit. Does that mean soy is the wonder bean and will cure diseases, prevent aging, and make you more beautiful? We have no idea. And we're not interested in delving deeper into the research that makes these claims. In our humble opinions based on research we trust, moderate consumption of organic soy products is safe. Do we eat ten servings a day? No. Do we take soy supplements? No. Do we add soy powders to our smoothies? No. Do we use soy as a wonder food or drug? No. But do we eat soy products? Yep.

We're not medical researchers or epidemiologists, so we'll

understand if our humble opinions don't mean shit to you. And even though countless doctors, medical researchers, and epidemiologists also feel moderate consumption of organic soy products is safe, their opinions may not mean shit to you, either. Good! You're questioning authority and taking matters into your own hands! If you're still not sure about soy, do your own research and decide for yourself, especially if you or your family members have thyroid problems or breast cancer. Knowledge is *self*-power. Kowtowing to your doctor without doing your own homework is just plain lazy. But be prepared to dig deep for the truth. Some pro-soy medical studies are paid for by the soy industry. Some anti-soy medical studies are paid for by the dairy and meat industries.

Remember, though, the majority of soybeans has been genetically modified and is laden with pesticides. So if you choose to eat soy products, you should definitely aim for organic. And use common sense, too. In general, the more processed a food is, the less wholesome it is for you. (Like eating an apple and a handful of nuts is healthier than eating an energy bar that has apple and nuts in it.) So whole soybeans, edamame, tofu, tempeh, and miso are more nutritious than other more highly processed soy foods. But if faced with eating chicken or soy chicken, meat or soy meat, cheese or soy cheese, we'd definitely choose the soy every time. (FYI: Many people find soy products to be excellent transitional foods for getting off meat and dairy products. Then, after a few months or even a year, they discontinue eating soy.) But also remember that it doesn't have to be either/or. You can abstain from eating animal products *and* soy and still have a healthy pregnancy. So long as you are eating a balance of fruits, veggies, whole grains, legumes, nuts, and seeds every day, and following doctors' orders for supplementing, you and your baby will thrive.

THE JOY OF FATS

One of the benefits of eschewing meat and dairy products is reducing your fat intake, which is a good thing. However, fats build and repair body tissue, manufacture hormones, and help transport vitamins. They're also vital for healthy fetal development! So be sure you're getting the good fats: Essential fatty acids, omega-3 and omega-6, can be found in dark, leafy green veggies, soybeans, avocados, nuts, seeds, and the oils of nuts and seeds. (Walnuts, flaxseeds, pumpkin seeds, and their oils are particularly good sources.[235]) So don't be a fat-free idiot—eat these foods daily.

But beware: Soy and nut allergies are among the most common. So if you, your husband, or anyone in your families have soy or nut allergies, check with your doctor before eating these foods.

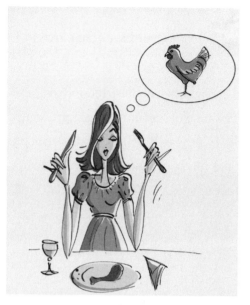

Chapter Seven

You (and Your Baby) Are What You Eat

There's a reason you've heard the adage, "You are what you eat," a million times . . . because it's true. Basically, everything you put in your mouth gets broken down and makes its way into your bloodstream, tissues, and organs. What doesn't come out in your pee or poo literally becomes a part of you. You are what you eat. Unfortunately, however, we've become detached from what we're eating because we've been eating the same things day after day, year after year, without a second thought. (Or, when we first started eating or drinking something we were under the impression it wasn't bad for us and we haven't revisited it since.) So now, drinking soda sweetened with chemicals seems normal and completely harmless. (It's neither.) Eating junk food laden with corn syrup and hydrogenated oils is totally common. (It shouldn't be.) And guzzling the milk from cow udders is considered vital. (Sheer madness.) We are completely removed from the fact that we are what we eat. So much that when we come across those who *don't* do these things because they *are* in touch with food and their bodies, we call them "health nuts!" The good news is, now that you're pregolas, you're forced to examine everything you put in your mouth. Everything you put in your mouth has either a positive or negative effect on you and your baby. When you really start to see food this way, nothing looks the same anymore. Which is a good thing, since most of us are either misinformed or deluded when it comes to food.

Most likely, when you first started reading the last two chapters, you thought *we* were deluded. Suggesting that pregnant women avoid meat and dairy products certainly goes against popular belief. But hopefully, by now, you realize we aren't deluded, and that we're actually just a couple of those "health nuts." If you aren't entirely convinced, we understand. It's a lot to swallow that much of what you've "known" your whole life is actually false or that your favorite foods are bad for you and your baby. So you have two choices: Remain deluded or live in the truth.

We know some of you *want* to live in the truth but you just can't buy what we're selling. It's tough to let go. Well, we're going to try and make it easier for you . . .

OLD MACDONALD HAD A MUCH DIFFERENT FARM

(This section will be familiar to those of you who read *Skinny Bitch*. We felt it warranted repeating.) Even knowing how abysmal the living conditions are for animals on factory farms, you cannot begin to imagine what the slaughter practices are like. "Humane" protocol calls for animals to be "stunned" before they are slaughtered. For cows, this means getting a metal bolt shot into the skull and then retracted. When done properly, using working equipment, this renders the cow unconscious. But time is money, and slaughterhouses operate at lightning speeds, some killing one animal every three seconds. Because thousands of frightened, struggling cows are not easy to stun, it is extremely common for a "stunner" to miss his mark.[236] Panicked hogs, also difficult to "hit," are stunned with an electric device. And if the jolt is too high, it bruises and bloodies the hogs' flesh (bad for business). Because business comes first on factory farms, the jolt is lowered, despite the fact that it doesn't properly stun the hogs.[237]

Stunned or not, cows and hogs are then "strung up" from the ceiling by a chain attached to their leg(s).[238] In theory, while they dangle there, they are supposed to be unconscious. But often they are fully conscious—struggling, screaming, and fearfully staring at the workers while they have their throats stabbed open.[239] Next, they travel along a "bleed rail," where they should bleed to death. But again, these large, frightened, struggling, conscious animals are difficult targets and the "stickers" (workers who cut their throats) don't always get a "good cut." Before cows can bleed to death, they are sent on their way to the "head-skinners," where the skin is sliced from their heads while they are still conscious.[240] Of course, this is excruciatingly painful, and the cows kick and struggle frantically. To avoid getting injured by the struggling animal, workers will sometimes sever the spinal cord with a knife blow to the back of the head. This paralyzes the animal below the neck so that the worker is safe. But these cows can still feel their skin being sliced away from their faces.[241] Next, their legs and head are chopped off, their entrails removed from their bodies, and then, finally, they are split in half. Often before hogs can bleed to death, they are dunked fully conscious into 140-degree Fahrenheit scalding water to remove the hair from their bodies.[242]

Egg-laying hens, because they are so overcrowded and stressed, frequently peck each other, so their beaks are literally chopped off their faces. Even though they currently comprise more than 95 percent of all land animals slaughtered for food, Congress exempted chickens (and turkeys) from the Humane Slaughter Act, so there is no requirement to stun them.[243] However, so the birds are immobilized when they arrive at the automated neck-slicer, in most slaughterhouses their heads are dragged through a water bath that has been electrically charged. This paralyzes the birds but does not render them unconcious.[244] They are snatched up, shackled upside down, and their throats are slashed by machine at the rate of thousands per hour.[245] Next, they are dunked in scalding water to loosen their feathers. Again, they are supposed to be dead at this point, but if the machine misses its mark, or the chickens haven't bled to death, they are boiled alive. Then they are placed into a series of machines that literally beat their feathers off of them, still alive and having just been boiled.[246] All the while, they are being handled like rubber toys: grabbed by their necks, feet, or wings and thrown around.

In egg-laying factories, male baby chicks are completely useless to farmers because they don't produce eggs. So workers snatch up chicks speeding by on a conveyer belt, quickly glance at their undersides, and then toss the "useless" males into the garbage. Yes. Literally. Millions of male baby chicks are piled on top of each other in garbage dumpsters, left to die. Or, more likely, they are tossed into macerators, and are ground up—alive.

In her book *Slaughterhouse*, Gail Eisnitz, chief investigator for the Humane Farming Association, interviewed dozens of slaughterhouse workers throughout the country. *Every single one* admitted to abusing animals or neglecting to report those who did.[247] The following are quotes from slaughterhouse workers taken from her book. (They are quite graphic and difficult to read, but we implore you to read each one. You and your baby are what you eat. Turning a blind eye will not erase what you're eating. Surely you can endure reading it if animals have to endure suffering it.)

"I seen them take those stunners—they're about as long as a yard stick—and shove it up the hog's ass. They do it with cows, too. And in their ears, their eyes, down their throat. They'll be squealing and they'll just shove it right down there."[248]

"Hogs get stressed out pretty easy. If you prod them too much they have heart attacks. If you get a hog in a chute that's had the shit prodded out of him and has a heart attack or refuses to move, you take a meat hook and hook it into his bunghole [anus]. You're dragging these hogs alive, and a lot of times the meat hook rips out of the bunghole. I've seen hams—thighs—completely ripped open. I've also seen intestines come out. If the hog collapses near the front of the chute, you shove the meat hook into his cheek and drag him forward."[249] "Or in their mouth. The roof of their mouth. And they're still alive."[250]

"Pigs on the kill floor have come up and nuzzled me like a puppy. Two minutes later I had to kill them—beat them to death with a pipe."[251]

"These hogs get up to the scalding tank, hit the water and start screaming and kicking. Sometimes they thrash so much they kick water out of the tank. . . . Sooner or later they drown. There's a rotating arm that pushes them under, no chance for them to get out. I'm not sure if they burn to death before they drown, but it takes them a couple of minutes to stop thrashing."[252]

"Sometimes I grab it [a hog] by the ear and stick it right through the eye. I'm not just taking its eye out, I'll go all the way to the hilt, right up through the brain, and wiggle the knife."[253]

"I could tell you horror stories about cattle getting their heads stuck under the gate guards, and the only way you can get it out is to cut their heads off while they're still alive."[254]

"I've seen live animals shackled, hoisted, stuck, and skinned. Too many to count, too many to remember. It's just a process that's continually there. I've seen shackled beef looking around before they've been stuck. I've seen hogs [that are supposed to be lying down] on the bleeding conveyor get up after they've been stuck. I've seen hogs in the scalding tub trying to swim."[255]

"I seen guys take broomsticks and stick it up the cow's behind, screwing them with a broom."[256]

"I've drug cows till their bones start breaking, while they were still alive. Bringing them around the corner and they get stuck up in the doorway, just pull them till their hide be ripped, till the blood just drip on the steel and concrete. Breaking their legs. . . . And the cow be crying with its tongue stuck out. They pull him till his neck just pop."[257]

"One time I took my knife—it's sharp enough—and I sliced off the end of a hog's nose, just like a piece of bologna. The hog went crazy for a few seconds. Then it just sat there looking kind of stupid. So I took a handful of salt brine and ground it into his nose. Now that hog really went nuts, pushing its nose all over the place. I still had a bunch of salt left in my hand—I was wearing a rubber glove—and I stuck the salt right up the hog's ass. The poor hog didn't know whether to shit or go blind."[258]

"Nobody knows who's responsible for correcting animal abuse at the plant. The USDA does zilch."[259]

Eisnitz chronicled the constant failure of U.S. Department of Agriculture inspectors to stop this abuse and their willingness to look the other way. In addition, she exposed the USDA's blatant tolerance for allowing contaminated meat into the human food supply. Think about it. *Ten billion* animals a year! Do you think the USDA has enough inspectors to supervise the humane and safe slaughter of *ten billion* animals a year? Of course the inspectors tolerate abuse and contaminated meat.

Imagine the kind of person who would have a job that entailed witnessing the slaughter of thousands of innocent animals every day. Even if every single inspector did a good job (they don't), the factory workers can easily bypass the system. Eisnitz interviewed one worker from a horse slaughterhouse, who said, "Might be part of him's [a contaminated horse] bad, might be the pneumonia's traveled everywhere. I'd drag him back, and my boss would tell me to cut the hindquarters off and bring him into the cooler. The meat's supposed to be condemned, but still you'd cut it up and bag it." When Eisnitz asked, "But don't they have to be stamped 'USDA inspected'?" he responded, "He [his boss] got the stamper. He can stamp it himself when the doc leaves.... You take a condemned horse, skin him, cut him up, sell the meat.... We've sold it as beef."[260] According to one former Perdue worker, the poultry plants are filthy. She said there were flies, rats, and 5-inch long flying cockroaches covering the walls and floors. [261] Believe it or not, it gets worse: "After they are hung, sometimes the chickens fall off into the drain that runs down the middle of the line. This is where roaches, intestines, diseased parts, fecal contamination, and blood are washed down. Workers [vomit] into the drain.... Employees are constantly chewing and spitting out snuff and tobacco on the floor... sometimes they have to relieve themselves on the floor.... The Perdue supervisors told us to take the fallen chickens out of the drain and send them down the line."[262] A USDA inspector said of the cockroaches, "One time we shined a flashlight into a hole they were crawling in and out, and they were so thick it was like maggots, you couldn't even see the surface."[263] A worker at another poultry plant said, "Every day, I saw black chicken, green chicken, chicken that stank, and chicken with feces on it. Chicken like this is supposed to be thrown away, but instead it would be sent down the line to be processed."[264] Another worker at another plant said, "I personally have seen rotten meat—you can tell by the odor. This rotten meat is mixed with the fresh meat and sold for baby food. We are asked to mix it with the fresh food, and this is the way it is sold. You can see the worms inside the meat."[265]

You and your baby are what you eat.

Animals hear the screaming and crying of other animals being slaughtered and are terrified. They know they are about to be killed and they are panic-stricken. When their young are taken from them, cows kick stall walls in rage and frustration and literally cry out with grief. Think of how you feel when you are angry, afraid, and grief-stricken. Bear in mind the physical feelings that accompany these emotions. These emotions—fear, grief, and rage—produce chemical changes in our bodies. They do the same to animals. Their blood pressures rise. Adrenaline courses through their bodies. You are eating high blood pressure, stress, and adrenaline. You are eating fear, grief, and rage. You are eating suffering, horror, and murder. You are eating cruelty. You and your baby are what you eat. You have a developing fetus growing inside you, feeding off what you eat. And you're eating fear, grief, and rage.

You want to know about "free-range" meat? Although a minuscule percentage of meat in the United States does come from free-range farms, how do you even know it is really free-range? Companies want us to believe that products labeled "free-range" or "free-roaming" are derived from animals that spent their short lives outdoors, enjoying sunshine, fresh air, and the company of other animals. But labels, other than "organic" on egg cartons, are not subject to any government regulations.[266] Because there are no agencies governing these claims, do you take the word of someone who makes a living on blood money? And even if the farm was free-range and humane, the animals are still being sent to horrific slaughter-houses. (An undercover video of a kosher slaughterhouse revealed animals suffering the same abuse and torture.)[267] Many animals don't even survive the transport from their factory, or free-range farms to slaughter. They often receive no food or water and no protection from the elements. Hundreds of thousands of animals are dead on arrival or too injured or sick to move. They don't get to stop for bathroom breaks, so the animals are forced to stand in their own urine and feces. In the wintertime, the animals' flesh and feet will actually freeze to the bottom and sides of the truck. So upon arrival, they are literally ripped away from the truck. One worker interviewed by Eisnitz said, "They freeze to that steel railing. They're still alive, and they'll hook a cable on it and pull it out, maybe pull a leg off."[268]

Yes, this information also applies to "free range" and "organic." "Free range" and "organic" do not mean cruelty-free. Cows who can no longer produce milk and hens who can no longer lay eggs are sent to slaughter. And they suffer immeasurably.

Assuming you started with a healthy animal (highly unlikely), you've now eaten hormones, pesticides, steroids, antibiotics, fear, grief, and rage. You and your baby are what you eat. But what if the animal wasn't healthy? Animals that are too sick or injured to walk were literally dragged to slaughter, one end of a chain attached to the animal, the other to a truck. The USDA still allowed these animals, referred to as "downers," to be slaughtered for human consumption until 2004! Finally, with the outbreak of more mad cow disease cases (a deadly and incurable disease that can be transmitted to humans through the consumption of cow flesh), they came to their senses. But consumer and animal rights groups had been lobbying to keep downers out of the food chain for more than a decade. In February 2008, long after downers were banned for consumption, the USDA ordered a recall of 143 million pounds of beef when undercover video footage revealed that downer cows were being slaughtered and processed for meat. Approximately 37 million pounds went to school lunch programs and other federal food programs, with the "great majority" of all the meat likely eaten before the recall, according to Dick Raymond, undersecretary of agriculture for food safety.[269] So knowing now what you do about factory farming, slaughterhouses, and the USDA, do you really believe downers will not make it into the food supply?

Do you believe that this was one isolated incident and that the rest of all the slaughterhouses operate differently? Yeah, we didn't think so. So in addition to all the other filth you're eating, you're also eating whatever illness the animal has. You and your baby are what you eat.

Let's make believe that all the animals killed for human consumption are healthy, happy, free of antibiotics, steroids, and pesticides and are humanely raised and slaughtered. Pretend you are eating "perfect meat." Great. But what exactly are you eating? Have you thought about this even once in the last decade, or ever? "Meat" is the decomposing, decaying, rotting flesh of a dead animal. As soon as an animal dies, it starts "breaking down." How long has passed between when the animal was slaughtered and the time you are eating it? It could be weeks, even months. You want to put a dead animal corpse—that has been rotting away for months—in your mouth? In your body? To nourish your developing baby? Because meat is muscle tissue, it oxidizes in an open environment and turns brown. So most meat markets will scrape off the brown parts to make it look more appealing. Another trick of the trade is using tinted lighting in open meat cases to enhance the meat's color.[270] Restaurants and ranchers might call their meat "aged to perfection," but no matter how you slice it, it's still a putrefying corpse. You and your baby are what you eat.

Being a mom means being compassionate and caring. Not just toward your own baby, but in general. Just because you can't see what's happening doesn't mean it doesn't exist. Every time you have a craving for meat or dairy, remember what goes on inside every farm, slaughterhouse, and processing plant. Paul McCartney's late wife, Linda McCartney, said it best: "If slaughterhouses had glass walls, we'd all be vegetarians."[271]

Now, some of you may be ready to explode. Certainly, when you bought this book, the last thing you expected is a chapter on factory farming and slaughter practices, and to be told that you should stop eating animals. But just because you didn't expect it or because it goes against what you've believed your whole life, it doesn't make the information any less accurate or valuable. Simmer down. Step back for a second. Ask yourself why you're angry. Wait sixty seconds. Now ask yourself again—usually the first time you're not able to see the truth. Chances are you're angry because we've revealed a huge pile of shit that you didn't want to see. You were perfectly happy eating burgers and chicken and eggs and cheese and bacon, and the last thing you wanted was to know exactly what you were eating all these years. You were perfectly happy thinking these foods were healthy, or at least "okay in moderation." You were perfectly happy not knowing just how cruel the meat and dairy industries are and how much suffering you were directly contributing to. Now that you know all this, you won't be able to be "perfectly happy" anymore without feeling repulsed, sickened, or guilty. Now that you know all this, you'll never be able to look at food the same way. Now that you know all this, you might actually have to change! Rather than change, some of you would prefer to numb out, hate us, or hold on to your old, unhealthy ways. For the sake of your unborn baby, we truly hope you'll embrace this change. But even more important, for yourselves, we hope you'll take it on. Because we both know from experience that abstaining from animal products is the best thing you can do for yourself.

If you absolutely cannot, will not, dare not believe what we're saying about meat and dairy, or you simply don't want to stop eating these foods—fine. Just don't throw the baby out with the bathwater! You know there's other useful information in this book. So don't use this as an excuse to dismiss everything else you've learned since you started reading it. Just ignore the stuff you simply can't abide by and incorporate what you can. No need be a drama queen about the whole thing.

If you're *completely* on board with us now, you are officially *vegan*, someone who doesn't eat any animal products. No meat, chicken, pork, fish, eggs, milk, cheese, or butter. Your husband will be thrilled. Ha! Or not. A lot of men think we're designed to eat meat. A lot of men are stupid. So this little section's for them:

Men, before you start spouting off information you've been brainwashed with about evolution and the food chain, read on. Yes, humans have a high level of intelligence. Yes, we created weapons for hunting and fire for cooking. Yes, we found a way to mass-produce animals for consumption. However, if you study animals in the wild, you will note that they do not rely on anything other than their natural hunting ability, speed, strength, claws, teeth, and jaws. They have no tools or weapons. Now look at yourself. Look at your flimsy fingernails in comparison to an eagle's talons. Look at your flat, blunt teeth compared with a lion's fangs. Compare your speed and agility to that of a tiger. Compare the strength of your jaw to a wolf's. Imagine yourself trying to run after an animal, catch it, and kill it using your bare hands, fingernails, teeth, and jaws. Not only would you look ridiculous, but you'd probably get your ass kicked, too. And even if you were successful, envision yourself eating the kill without the aid of an oven and silverware.[272] Yes, the human brain allows us to stay removed from the process of hunting. But does this mean we are "evolved" and "intelligent" and should be eating animal flesh just because we can? Man's brain and "intelligence" also created alcohol, cigarettes, and drugs. Should we drink, smoke, and use just because we can?

Many meat eaters credit eating meat for our evolution from cavemen into what we are now. Even if this were the case and eating meat did help us to evolve, look at what we evolved *from*. We looked like apes and had massive heads, strong jaws, and brute strength. (And we were covered in hair from head to toe!) Maybe, back then, we were supposed to eat meat. But the last time we checked, we aren't cavemen anymore.

The second we put food in our mouths, the digestion process begins, thanks to our saliva. Guess what? Our alkaline saliva is not meant to break down animal flesh; carnivores have acid saliva, perfectly designed for the task. And hydrochloric acid, essential for digesting carcass, is secreted in very small amounts in our stomachs. However, the stomachs of carnivores have ten times more hydrochloric acid than ours. Our enzymes, digestive tracts, and organs are all different from those found in carnivores. Like it or not, our kidneys, colon, and liver are ill-equipped to process animal flesh. Compared with carnivores, our intestines are very long, so food that doesn't get adequately processed becomes clogged in our intestines. Animals quickly pass food through their digestive systems, but we have food rotting, decomposing, and putrefying in our intestinal tracts and colons, hence the need for colonics. You don't see many tigers getting colonics, do you? You do see them napping, though. Even though their bodies are designed to digest meat, animals generally sleep all day while doing so because it is such a taxing process. Genetically and structurally, we are designed to thrive on plant foods.[273] Sorry, fellas. You can go back to your remote controls, now.

All kidding aside, it is absolutely safe for pregnant women to be vegetarian or vegan. The American Academy of Pediatrics, the National Academy of Sciences, and the American Medical Association have all spoken in favor of veg pregnancies.[274] The American Dietetic Association states, "Well-planned vegan and other types of vegetarian diets are appropriate for all stages of the life cycle, including during pregnancy, lactation, infancy, childhood, and adolescence."[275] In fact, it's not only *safe,* it's likely *safer* to have a veg pregnancy.

- According to the National Center for Health Statistics, one out of three babies is born by C-section in the United States.[276] Yikes! In Tennessee, there is a large vegan community known as The Farm. A study of 1,700 vegan mothers-to-be revealed that only one in one hundred women delivered by C-section![277]

- And in twenty years, there was only one case of preeclampsia,[278] compared with the national average, which is 10 percent![279] Magnesium deficiency is associated with eclampisa. As reported in the *European Journal of Clinical Nutrition*, researchers found that women adhering to plant-based diets had better magnesium levels and fewer magnesium deficiency-related problems than their meat-eating counterparts.[280]

- The Institute of Medicine found that pregnant vegetarians are more likely to have adequate vitamin A intake than pregnant meat-eaters. It just so happens that vitamin A deficiencies have been linked to higher rates of miscarriage![281]

- According to the *New England Journal of Medicine*, vegan moms had dramatically lower levels of toxic chemicals in their breast milk compared with other lactating moms. In fact, the *highest* level of the vegan moms was still lower than the *lowest* level of the meat-eating moms! The difference was staggering: The breast milk of the veg moms had levels of contamination only 1 to 2 percent as great the others![282]

It's not just safe for mothers-to-be to be vegans. According to the medical journal, *Pediatrics in Review*, "Multiple experts have concluded independently that vegan diets can be followed safely by infants and children without compromise of nutrition or growth and with some notable health benefits." Even Dr. Benjamin Spock, the most esteemed pediatrician of all time, recommended children be raised vegan. His book, *Dr. Spock's Baby and Child Care*, is literally one of the best-selling books of all time.[283] In his seventh edition, he changed his tune after decades and began advocating a plant-based diet.[284]

So why all the negativity around veganism? Why does it have such a bad rap? Typically, anything out of the ordinary or anything that people don't fully understand can be frowned upon. Collectively, the world develops a negative opinion about it. We influence one another to share this opinion, and we actually ridicule those who don't. And in this day and age, we have the media telling us what's good and bad, in and out, right and wrong. And the media's driven by the collective "cool." Poor veganism barely stood a chance. In 2007, a couple was sentenced to life in prison for starving their newborn son to death. They were vegans. You can likely remember reading about it and seeing it on the news. You probably don't remember that the prosecuting attorney did not in any way condemn veganism. He said, "The vegan diet is fine. These parents lied about what they fed him. He was just not fed enough."[285] Sadly, this wasn't the first case of vegan parents starving or neglecting their children. In 2003, a vegan couple in New York was accused of starving their baby. In both cases, people nationwide hurled hate, anger, and rage at vegetarianism, calling it "dangerous," "radical," and "child abuse." What these parents did was wrong. It was irresponsible, stupid, senseless, and devastating. They starved their children. And they were vegans. Does it mean veganism is dangerous? Does it mean vegans are cruel? Does it mean vegans are crazy? No. It means that these individuals are sick. It just so happens they are vegan—much to the chagrin of the millions of normal vegan parents all over the world. When meat-eating, milk-drinking parents starve their children to death, the headlines don't sensationalize their dietary choices. Because those parents are "normal" in that regard.

We've both been vegan for years, and we've both been studying nutrition for years. Unsurprisingly, we've stumbled upon anti-veg information more than a few times. So when we heard about one particular study regarding fetal penis development, it piqued our curiosity but didn't raise our eyebrows too much. It was reported that pregnant vegetarians were more likely than pregnant meat-eaters to have sons with hypospadias. (Hypospadias is a condition, correctable by surgery, where the opening of the penis is on the underside instead of the tip.)[286] Sounds scary, yes. But after reading the study ourselves and consulting with multiple doctors, epidemiologists, and other health experts, we felt less afraid and more annoyed. For starters, there were only seven boys born to vegetarian moms who had the condition.[287] Seven. Not a very significant number to base a hypothesis on. Especially since millions of babies have been born to vegetarian women around the world for decades, and not one other study exists to support the claim. Additionally, in the study, there were other factors found to affect the likelihood of hypospadias—iron supplementation and incidence of flu during the first trimester.[288] Yet the study was titled, "Maternal vegetarian diet in pregnancy linked to hypospadias." Not only does veg-bashing make for a more sensational headline than flu- or iron supplementation-bashing, but it also betters the chances of receiving future funding for subsequent studies. Especially given that data collection was funded in part by the Meat and Livestock Commission.[289]

So here we are, all squawking that vegetarian men grow boobs and other stupid shit like that. But the truth is, well-planned vegetarian and vegan diets are perfectly safe for pregnant women and babies alike.

Not only that, but plant-based diets are better for the environment. Now that you're having children, can you please start caring about the environment? If you don't, they might not have an ozone left to play in! Every environmentalist knows that factory farming is completely destroying the planet. As ridiculous as it sounds, the methane resulting from the burps and farts of ten billion animals a year is directly responsible for global warming.[290] Believe it or not, according to the United Nations Food and Agriculture Organization, raising animals for food causes more greenhouse gas emissions than cars![291] This warrants repeating: Raising animals for food causes more greenhouse gas emissions than cars. In addition, the urine and feces are polluting and contaminating soil and water all over the world. According to the Environmental Protection Agency, they are the largest polluters of U.S. waterways.[292] Moreover, the amount of land, food, water, and energy used to raise farm animals for food could actually be used to grow food for *all of the starving people in the world.*[293] That's right—you being vegan is actually a step toward ending world hunger. Talk about starting your baby's life off with some good-ass karma!

You and your baby are what you eat.

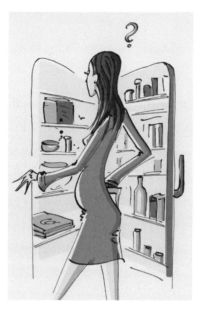

Chapter Eight
What the Hell to Eat

So you shouldn't eat cows, chickens, pigs, fish, milk, cheese, or eggs. So what the hell should you eat? Pretty much everything else: fruits, vegetables, legumes, nuts, seeds, and whole grains. Deep down, you've known all along that these foods are best for you; now it's time to get back on track. Our diets have strayed so far off course from where they belong; we've allowed meat to take center stage, with grains and vegetables playing supporting roles. Wrong, wrong, wrong. There is a plethora of great-tasting, healthy, wholesome foods that you've likely been neglecting for years. Well, those days are over. Get back to the basics and enjoy all these excellent foods you forgot about. You've got a baby to think about!

Remember in grade-school when you learned about photosynthesis? Plants store the sun's energy, which we receive by eating them. Picture the light energy from the sun beaming down to the vegetables and fruits, and as you eat those foods, imagine that energy being transmitted into your body and your baby's. Our nervous systems are maintained and stimulated by this light. What an amazing gift from nature—to be able to eat such pure foods that give our bodies and babies so much!

However, be advised, all fruits and vegetables are not created equal. Plants need vitamins and minerals to function and grow properly. When they are sprayed with pesticides and grown in chemically treated soil, they won't absorb all the proper nutrients. This results in a loss of enzymes. So, organic fruits and vegetables—ones that have been grown in pure, untreated soil and without pesticides—have far more enzymes[294] and nutrients[295] than their conventionally grown counterparts. You and your baby are what you eat.

Any scientist can tell you that food has an "energy" or "life" to it. Anyone with common sense can tell you that eating a live, fresh fruit is healthier than eating a cooked, canned, preserved one. Why? Because this "life" comes from the plant's energy, nutrients, phytochemicals, and enzymes. Enzymes are living biochemical factors that we need to survive. They are critical for digestion, breathing, reproduction, and the functioning of DNA and RNA. They also help repair and heal our organs, detoxify our bodies, carry out our nerve impulses, and help us think.

There are three types of enzymes: metabolic, digestive, and food. Fortunately, we produce our own metabolic enzymes, which run the whole body, maintain our health, and defend us from illness and infection. We also produce digestive enzymes. But our own enzyme supplies are limited. So to continue healthy bodily functions, we need to supplement with food. When we eat, our bodies release digestive enzymes to break down the food. If we eat foods devoid of enzymes, such as meat, processed food, and even just overcooked food (high temperatures destroy enzymes), our bodies have to work much harder.[296] Harder work means using more of our precious enzymes. Over time, this can result in an enlargement of the digestive organs and the endocrine glands.[297] This lack of enzymes can also cause a disruption in the body's ability to make enough metabolic enzymes. But when we eat foods high in enzymes, such as fruits, salad, or lightly steamed veggies, we get an enzyme boost along with the meal, so our bodies don't have to work so hard. There is no greater defender of our bodies than enzymes. When not in use for digestion, enzymes are busy repairing and cleaning our bodies.[298] So don't go throwing your enzymes away on junk!

So how do we get these enzymes into our bodies? We just need to make the following foods part of our daily diets: fruits, raw or lightly steamed vegetables, raw nuts and seeds, sea vegetables (like kelp, seaweeds, etc.), and legumes.

Don't worry if you've never eaten this way before. We've compiled a few food lists to help you. And if your grocery store doesn't carry something you see on our lists, remember, ask for it! Lots of places are happy to accommodate customer requests. But if you still can't find the foods we list here, don't get your panties in a bunch. By the time you're done reading the book, you'll know how to shop and what to look for in ingredients.

BREAKFAST FOOD LIST

(R) found in refrigerator section
(F) found in freezer section

Arrowhead Mills: Organic Blue Corn Pancake
   and Waffle Mix
Arrowhead Mills: Organic Whole Grain Pancake
   and Waffle Mix
Food for Life: Ezekiel 4:9 Cereal
Nature's Path: Optimum Slim Cereal
Nature's Path: Optimum Power Breakfast Cereal
Health Valley: Organic Raisin Bran Flakes
Health Valley: Organic Oat Bran Flakes with Raisins
Old Wessex Ltd.: Irish-Style Oatmeal
Old Wessex Ltd.: 5-Grain Cereal
Nature's Path: Organic Instant Hot Maple Nut Oatmeal
Nature's Path: Organic Manna Breads (F)
Ancient Harvest: Organic Quinoa Flakes
Rice Dream: Original Enriched Rice Milk
Original EdenSoy: Organic Soymilk
Original EdenBlend: Rice & Soy Beverage
House: Tofu Steak (R)
Whole Soy & Co.: Creamy Cultured Soy (yogurt) (R)
So Delicious: Creamy Cultured Soy (yogurt) (R)
So Delicious: Coconut Milk Yogurt (R)
Silk: Cultured Soy (yogurt) (R)
Amy's: Organic Tofu Scramble (F)

Azna Gluten-Free (www.aznaglutenfree.com)**:** Waffles (F)
Van's: All-Natural Organic Original Waffles (F)
Lifestream: Mesa Sunrise Toaster Waffles
French Meadow Bakery: Men's Bread
French Meadow Bakery: Healthy Hemp Sprouted Bread
French Meadow Bakery: Brown Rice Bread
Fabe's All Natural Bakery: Vegan Muffins (F)
Zen Bakery: Muffins (R)
Zen Bakery: Cinnamon Raisin Rolls (R)
Whole Foods: Organic English Muffins (R)
Food for Life: Ezekiel 4:9 Sprouted Grain Bagels (F)
Tofutti: Better Than Cream Cheese (R)
   (the kind without hydrogenated oils)
Lightlife: Smart Bacon (R)
Lightlife: Gimme Lean! Sausage Style (R)
organic fruit

LUNCH FOOD LIST

Food for Life: Ezekiel 4:9 bread (F) (or bakery/bread aisle)
Arrowhead Mills: Organic Valencia Peanut Butter
MaraNatha: Organic Raw Almond Butter
I.M. Healthy: SoyNut Butter
Bionaturae: organic fruit spreads
Natural Touch: Tuno (faux tuna)
Morningstar Farms: Tuno
Amy's: All-American Burger (F)
Amy's: California Burger (F)

Amy's: Texas Burger (F)
Gardenburger: Flame-Grilled Burgers (F)
Gardenburger: Flame-Grilled Chik'n (F)
Whole Foods Bakehouse: Organic Burger Buns
Tofurkey: Deli Slices
Yves: Veggie Bologna (R)
Yves: Veggie Turkey (R)
Yves: Veggie Salami (R)
Follow Your Heart: Vegan Gourmet Cheese Alternative (R)
Sheese (www.blackduckimports.com)**:** Vegan cheeses
    and cream cheeses (R)
Teese (www.teesecheese.com)**:** Vegan Cheese (R)
Earthbound Farm: Organic Salad Greens (R)
Fantastic Foods: Tabouli
Fantastic Foods: Organic Whole Wheat Couscous
Fantastic Carb 'Tastic Soup: Vegetarian Chicken Gumbo
Fantastic Carb 'Tastic Soup: Shiitake Mushroom
Fantastic Big Soup: Five Bean
Fantastic Big Soup: Country Lentil
Amy's Organic Soups: Black Bean Vegetable
Amy's Organic Soups: Butternut Squash
Amy's Organic Soups: Lentil Vegetable
Amy's Organic Soups: Chunky Vegetable
Amy's: Organic Chili
Health Valley: Organic Split Pea Soup
Health Valley: Organic Lentil Soup
Health Valley: Organic Black Bean Soup
Imagine: Organic Vegetable Broth

Imagine: Organic No-Chicken Broth
Pacific: Organic Vegetable Broth
organic vegetables

DINNER FOOD LIST

Health Best 100% Organic: Red Lentils
Health Best 100% Organic: Green Lentils
Health Best 100% Organic: Barley
Health Best 100% Organic: Split Peas
Health Best 100% Organic: Amaranth
Arrowhead Mills: Organic Whole Millet
Lundberg Family Farms: Organic Short Grain Brown Rice
Lundberg Family Farms: Organic Brown Rice Pasta
DeBoles: Organic Whole Wheat Pasta
Ancient Harvest: Organic Quinoa Supergrain Pasta
Eddie's Spaghetti: Organic Vegetable Pasta
Pastariso: Organic Brown Rice Fettuccine
Pastariso: Organic Brown Rice Elbow Macaroni
Rising Moon Organics: Spinach Florentine Ravioli
    with Tofu (F)
Chef Nikola's Kitchen: Roasted Eggplant in Herbed
    Balsamic Sauce (F)
Amy's Organic: Asian Noodle Stir-Fry (F)
Amy's Organic: Thai Stir-Fry (F)
Amy's: Roasted Vegetable Pizza (no cheese) (F)
Nate's: Meatless Meatballs (F)
Health Is Wealth: Buffalo Wings (F)

Health Is Wealth: Chicken-Free Patties (F)
Health Is Wealth: Chicken-Free Nuggets (F)
Tofurkey: Tofurkey Dinner (F)
Gloria's Kitchen: assorted vegan prepared entrees (F)
Lightlife: Organic Tempeh (R)
Lightlife: Smart Ground (ground "meat") (F)
Nasoya: Organic Tofu (R)
White Wave: Chicken-Style Seitan (R)
Lightlife: Smart Dogs (R)
Yves: Veggie Dogs (R)
Rudi's Organic Bakery: White Hot Dog Rolls
Now & Zen: UnChicken (R)
Now & Zen: UnSteak (R)
Yves: Veggie Ground Round Mexican
    (Mexican-style ground "meat") (F)
Azna Gluten-Free (www.aznaglutenfree.com): Pizza Dough (F)
Bearitos: Taco Shells
Garden of Eatin': Blue Corn Taco Shells
Alvarado St. Bakery: Organic Sprouted Wheat Tortillas
organic vegetables

(Obviously, the foods on the lunch and dinner lists can be interchanged.)

We didn't forget about the snacks and treats we promised you. Yes, there are "acceptable" junk foods. No, you shouldn't gorge on them.

ACCEPTABLE JUNK FOOD, SNACKS & DESSERTS

Dr. Cow (www.dr-cow.com)**:** Tree Nut Cheese

Sunflour Baking Company: all products

365: Organic Chocolate Soymilk

Whole Foods: Organic Date Coconut Rolls

Barbara's Bakery: organic graham crackers

Dagoba: organic dark chocolate bars

Uncle Eddie's: vegan cookies

Organica Foods: vegan cookies

Fabe's All Natural Bakery: vegan cookies, pies, cakes, and macaroons

Laura's Wholesome Junk Food: Bitelettes (cookies)

Nutrilicious Natural Bakery: Donut Holes

MI-DEL: Vanilla Snaps

Country Choice: Certified Organic Sandwich Cremes

Back to Nature: Classic Creme Sandwich Cookies

Back to Nature: Chocolate & Mint Creme Sandwich Cookies

Chocolove: Belgian dark chocolate

Endangered Species: dark chocolate bars

Tropical Source: rice crisp dark chocolate

Ecco Bella: Health by Chocolate

Raw Balance (www.rawbalance.com)**:** Carobelles (R)

Gertrude & Bronner's Magic: Alpsnack

LäraBar: all flavors

Terra: exotic vegetable chips original

Terra: spiced sweet potato chips

Maine Coast Sea Vegetables: Sea Chips
Garden of Eatin': Sunny Blues (tortilla chips with
    sunflower seeds)
Guiltless Gourmet: Yellow Corn Baked Chips
Kettle Organic Tortilla Chips: Sesame Blue Moons
Veggie Stix: Shoestring Potato Sticks
Robert's American Gourmet: Tings, Spicy Tings, Veggie Booty
Newman's Own: Organic Salted Round Pretzels
Koyo Organic Rice Cakes: Dulse
Koyo Organic Rice Cakes: Mixed Grain
Nature's Path: Tamari Flax Crackers
Back to Nature: Classic Rounds
Soy Dream: non-dairy frozen desserts (F)
So Delicious: non-dairy frozen desserts (F)
Soy Delicious: Li'l Buddies ("ice cream" sandwiches) (F)
Purely Decadent: non-dairy frozen dessert (F)
Purely Decadent: coconut milk non-dairy frozen dessert (F)
Azna Gluten-Free (www.aznaglutenfree.com)**:** cinnamon
    rolls, scones (F)
Organic fruit, organic vegetables, organic nuts & seeds

Don't worry about the little odds and ends. We've thought of everything.

CONDIMENTS, BAKING SUPPLIES & MISCELLANEOUS

Parma: Vegan Parmesan
Earth Balance: Natural Buttery Spread (R)
Soy Garden: Natural Buttery Spread (R)
Follow Your Heart: Vegenaise (mayonnaise substitute) (R)
Nasoya: Nayonaise
Muir Glen: Organic Ketchup
Westbrae: Natural Ketchup
Whole Kids: Organic Yellow Mustard
Spectrum Naturals: Organic Sesame Oil
Spectrum Naturals: Organic Canola Oil
Spectrum Naturals: Organic Extra Virgin Olive Oil
MaraNatha: Organic Raw Tahini
Bragg Liquid Aminos: All-Purpose Seasoning (soy sauce substitute)
Sea Seasonings: Organic Kelp Granules With Cayenne
Annie's Naturals: Goddess Dressing
OrganicVille: Sesame Tamari Organic Vinaigrette
The Wizard's: Organic Original Vegetarian Worcestershire Sauce
Essential Living Foods: Organic Agave Nectar Or Syrup
Shady Maple Farms: Certified Organic Pure Maple Syrup

Sugar in the Raw: Turbinado Sugar from Natural Cane
Florida Crystals: Organic Cane Sugar
Wholesome Sweeteners: Organic Sucanat
Hain Pure Foods: Organic Brown Sugar
Stevita Company Inc.: Stevia Spoonable
Dr. Oetker Organics: Chocolate Cake Mix
Dr. Oetker Organics: Vanilla Cake Mix
Dr. Oetker Organics: Chocolate Icing Mix
Dr. Oetker Organics: Vanilla Icing Mix
Dr. Oetker Organics: Chocolate Chip Cookie Mix
Ener-G: Egg Replacer
Chatfield's Carob & Compliments: Dairy-Free Carob
   Morsels
Sunspire: Grain-Sweetened Chocolate Chips
Arrowhead Mills: Organic Oat Flour
Arrowhead Mills: Organic Whole Wheat Flour
Arrowhead Mills: Organic Spelt Flour
Arrowhead Mills: Organic Brown Rice Flour
Arrowhead Mills: Organic Blue Corn Meal
Arrowhead Mills: Organic Yellow Corn Meal
Arrowhead Mills: Organic Flax Seeds
Udo's: DHA Oil Blend

Still a little confused or overwhelmed? Jeesh! Do we have to do everything for you? Here are four weeks' worth of menus for you to use as a guide:

WEEK ONE

Monday

Breakfast: Two pieces wholegrain toast with almond butter and banana slices, vanilla soy yogurt with blueberries, and calcium-fortified orange juice.

Snack: Hummus with carrots and celery.

Lunch: Grilled portobello mushroom sandwich with red bell pepper pesto, lettuce, tomatoes, and soy cheese on a wholegrain bun. Served with a small bowl of broccoli bisque soup.

Snack: Fruit salad.

Dinner: Vegan three-bean Southwest tempeh chili with corn, carrots and kale. Served with corn muffins and a glass of calcium-fortified rice milk.

Tuesday

Breakfast: Granola with strawberries and calcium-fortified soymilk served with a piece of cantaloupe and calcium-fortified orange juice.

Snack: Flaxseed crackers with sundried tomato pâté and a green apple.

Lunch: Leftover chili and corn muffin served with a mixed green salad with cucumbers and beets.

Snack: Raw almonds and cashews and a mixed-berry smoothie.

Dinner: Vegetable lasagna with tofu, eggplant, red peppers, and zucchini and wholegrain garlic bread.

Wednesday

Breakfast: Wholegrain cinnamon French toast (dip it in rice milk instead of egg batter) served with raspberries and bananas and calcium-fortified orange juice.

Snack: Banana walnut bread with soy cream cheese and low-sodium vegetable juice.

Lunch: Lentil burger with avocado slices, lettuce, and tomato on a wholegrain bun served with dill potato salad.

Snack: A sliced apple served with peanut butter and sun-flower seeds and a glass of almond milk.

Dinner: Shepherd's pie made with soy meat crumbles, mashed potatoes, carrots, and peas served with a tossed salad with tomatoes and herbs.

Thursday

Breakfast: Nutty oatmeal made with calcium-fortified rice milk, blueberries, and raspberries and sprinkled with ground flaxseeds and almonds. Serve with grapefruit juice.

Snack: Soy yogurt and an orange.

Lunch: Grilled tempeh Rueben with avocado slices served on wholegrain bread with a side of tabbouleh.

Snack: Steamed edamame.

Dinner: Brown rice with sautéed spinach, garlic, asparagus, and pine nuts served with garlic whole-wheat rosemary bread.

Friday

Breakfast: Tofu scramble with zucchini, mushrooms, and leeks served with fresh squeezed apple/carrot juice, a wholegrain English muffin, and 100 percent fruit jam.

Snack: An orange, a handful of figs, and a handful of raw Brazil nuts.

Lunch: Seitan sloppy Joes on a wholegrain sesame-seed roll with a carrot, beet, and sunflower seed salad.

Snack: Fruit salad sprinkled with wheat germ.

Dinner: Brown rice, broccoli, and lentil-stuffed red peppers served with a salad of spinach, walnuts, and faux feta and a glass of calcium-fortified soymilk.

Saturday

Breakfast: Nutty oatmeal made with calcium-fortified rice milk with almonds, strawberries, and bananas served with calcium-fortified orange juice.

Snack: Soy yogurt with blueberries.

Lunch: Tofu sandwich with cilantro pesto and lettuce, tomatoes, and avocado slices on multi-grain bread served with a barley corn salad.

Snack: Trail mix with nuts and raisins and low-sodium
   vegetable juice.

Dinner: Moroccan-style tempeh with broccoli and mustard
   greens served with couscous pilaf and whole-wheat
   pita chips.

Sunday

Breakfast: Raspberry bran muffin with soy butter, veggie
   sausage, a grapefruit, and calcium-fortified orange juice.

Snack: Fruit salad sprinkled with wheat germ and
   sunflower seeds.

Lunch: Split pea soup, arugula salad with beets, daikon and
   carrots, and a wholegrain roll.

Snack: Peanut butter and jelly (100 percent fruit) sandwich
   and a glass of calcium-fortified rice milk.

Dinner: Thai tofu stir-fry with bok choy, snow peas, and
   whole-wheat soba noodles.

WEEK TWO

Monday

Breakfast: Soy bacon, lettuce, tomato, and avocado on
   wholegrain bread and calcium-fortified rice milk.

Snack: Fruit salad sprinkled with ground flaxseeds and a
   handful of walnuts and almonds.

Lunch: Grilled eggplant, red pepper, zucchini, and hummus, whole-wheat pita pockets, and a small mixed-green salad.

Snack: Macadamia coconut muffin and a glass of calcium-fortified orange juice.

Dinner: Mexican three-bean and seitan casserole with carrots and jicama, served with quinoa and a corn muffin.

Tuesday

Breakfast: Tofu, spinach and mushroom "quiche" with a raspberry flaxseed muffin and fresh-squeezed apple/ carrot/ beet juice.

Snack: Fruit salad sprinkled with chopped walnuts and wheat germ.

Lunch: Potato, fennel, and leek soup served with a chickpea salad with artichokes, parsley, and sundried tomatoes.

Snack: Steamed broccoli and asparagus tips with garlic and olive oil and a wholegrain roll with soy butter.

Dinner: Pumpkin, sage, and pecan ravioli with soy butter, steamed kale and mustard greens, served with a glass of calcium-fortified soymilk.

Wednesday

Breakfast: Granola with calcium-fortified rice milk, dates,

figs, strawberries, and bananas and calcium-fortified
orange juice.

Snack: Edamame.

Lunch: BBQ tofu salad with raw carrots, celery, and red
peppers served with seeded wholegrain bread.

Snack: Almond butter and banana sandwich and chocolate
calcium-fortified soymilk.

Dinner: Herbed polenta with grilled zucchini and squash
served with steamed kale.

Thursday

Breakfast: Smoothie made with calcium-fortified rice milk,
soy yogurt, strawberries, and bananas served with cinnamon raisin walnut bread.

Snack: Flaxseed crackers with cauliflower spread.

Lunch: Minestrone soup and a multi-grain roll served with a
salad of spinach, pears, and walnuts.

Snack: Trail mix and calcium-fortified orange juice.

Dinner: Lentil and brown rice curry with potatoes, cabbage,
and broccoli.

Friday

Breakfast: Oatmeal made with almond milk, blueberries,
strawberries, and ground flaxseeds served with calcium-
fortified orange juice.

Snack: Mixed raw nuts and carrot/beet juice.

Lunch: Three-bean and quinoa salad with parsley, tomatoes, and green beans over mixed greens. Served with
a multi-grain roll.
Snack: Zucchini nut bread with soy butter and a peach.
Dinner: Collard greens, kale, and garlic with sautéed
tempeh and a baked sweet potato.

Saturday

Breakfast: Buckwheat blueberry pancakes, calcium-
fortified orange juice, and veggie sausage links.
Snack: Guacamole and hummus with sliced cucumbers and
carrots and vegetable juice.
Lunch: Chilled soba noodles with tofu, snow peas, and red
peppers in a peanut sesame sauce.
Snack: Mixed-berry smoothie made with soy yogurt served
with a handful of raw almonds.
Dinner: Mushroom and potato barley stew with wholegrain
rosemary bread.

Sunday

Breakfast: Flaxseed raisin bran cereal with calcium-fortified
soymilk and mixed berries served with pomegranate juice.
Snack: Apple slices with almond butter, banana slices, and
sunflower seeds.
Lunch: Butternut squash soup with a hummus and
veggie wrap.

Snack: White bean dip with pretzels and carrot/apple juice.

Dinner: Sautéed seitan with broccoli, asparagus, and mushroom gravy over whole-wheat couscous. Served with toasted multi-grain garlic bread.

WEEK THREE

Monday

Breakfast: Blueberry banana muffin, strawberry soy yogurt sprinkled with wheat germ, served with calcium-fortified orange juice.

Snack: Fruit salad with figs and raw cashews.

Lunch: Burrito with brown rice, black beans, avocado, and soy cheese with a tomato and jicama side salad.

Snack: Lentil walnut pâté with sesame rice crackers.

Dinner: Barley stew with carrots, lentils, wakame, and celery, served with rosemary potato bread.

Tuesday

Breakfast: Spinach, mushroom, and tomato tofu scramble with wholegrain toast and calcium-fortified orange juice.

Snack: Mixed nuts and dried fruit and apple/carrot/beet juice.

Lunch: Mediterranean platter with hummus, eggplant, grape leaves, peppers, olives, and tomatoes with whole-wheat pita bread.

Snack: A peanut butter–coated banana and a glass of
calcium-fortified chocolate rice milk.
Dinner: Polenta pie with kidney beans, white beans,
broccoli, and cabbage.

Wednesday

Breakfast: Oatmeal with calcium-fortified rice milk,
sunflower seeds, and mixed berries served with calcium-
fortified orange juice.
Snack: Trail mix and vegetable juice.
Lunch: Jasmine rice and red bean salad with corn, avo-
cado, tomato, and red pepper over steamed spinach.
Served with a wholegrain roll.
Snack: Banana walnut bread with soy cream cheese.
Dinner: Pistachio-crusted tempeh with black-eyed peas,
corn, collard greens, kale, and brown rice.

Thursday

Breakfast: Flaxseed raisin bran cereal with calcium-fortified
soymilk and strawberries and calcium-fortified orange
juice.
Snack: Fruit smoothie and a handful of cashews.
Lunch: Lentil soup with a small mixed-green salad.
Snack: Peanut butter and jelly (100 percent fruit) sandwich
and pomegranate juice.

Dinner: BBQ tempeh kabobs with grilled red peppers, onions, zucchini, and a side of jasmine rice, served with toasted pita chips.

Friday

Breakfast: Banana buckwheat pancakes with veggie sausage and calcium-fortified orange juice.

Snack: Fruit salad sprinkled with wheat germ and a handful of walnuts.

Lunch: Whole-wheat pasta salad with artichokes, parsley, sundried tomatoes, and olives and a glass of calcium-fortified soymilk.

Snack: Flaxseed crackers with guacamole and hummus and a carrot/apple juice.

Dinner: Miso soup and sautéed tofu, red peppers, and shitake mushrooms.

Saturday

Breakfast: Smoothie made with calcium-fortified almond milk, bananas, strawberries, wheat germ, and tahini and banana nut bread.

Snack: Blueberry soy yogurt with raisins.

Lunch: Roasted veggie quesadilla with avocado and soy cheese on a whole-wheat tortilla served with a small mixed-green salad.

Snack: Fruit salad and a handful of almonds.

Dinner: Cajun gumbo with black beans, barley, tempeh, carrots, and sweet potatoes served with broccoli and cornbread.

Sunday

Breakfast: Multi-grain cinnamon French toast with raspberries and calcium-fortified orange juice.

Snack: Blueberry soy yogurt with ground flaxseeds and wheat germ.

Lunch: Black bean and lentil burger with lettuce, tomato, and avocado on a wholegrain bun with potato salad.

Snack: Granola bar, a peach, and pomegranate juice.

Dinner: Whole-wheat spaghetti with "meat" balls and tomato sauce, served with garlic bread, a small mixed-green salad, and a glass of calcium-fortified soymilk.

WEEK FOUR

Monday

Breakfast: Oatmeal with calcium-fortified rice milk, almonds, sunflower seeds, and strawberries and fresh-squeezed grapefruit juice.

Snack: Fruit smoothie and a macadamia coconut muffin.

Lunch: Carrot and sweet potato soup with a side salad of adzuki beans, squash, and seaweed.

Snack: Trail mix and dates and carrot/beet juice.

Dinner: Seitan pot-pie with potatoes, peas, and broccoli and a small side salad with tomatoes and cucumbers.

Tuesday

Breakfast: Whole-wheat English muffin with almond butter, tahini, and bananas served with a slice of cantaloupe and calcium-fortified orange juice.

Snack: Edamame

Lunch: Veggie burger with sautéed mushrooms, avocado, lettuce, tomato, and onion on a wholegrain roll served with roasted sweet potato wedges and a glass of calcium-fortified rice milk.

Snack: Fruit salad sprinkled with wheat germ.

Dinner: Sesame-crusted tofu sticks with sautéed bok choy, shiitake mushrooms, and brown rice.

Wednesday

Breakfast: "Egg" sandwich made with tofu, melted soy cheese, and soy bacon on a whole-grain bagel, served with calcium-fortified orange juice.

Snack: Fruit smoothie and a handful of walnuts.

Lunch: Caesar salad with soy chicken strips and croutons.

Snack: Peanut butter and banana sandwich and a glass of calcium-fortified rice milk.

Dinner: Brown rice with sautéed Brussels sprouts, carrots, kale and white beans and a small mixed-green salad.

Thursday

Breakfast: Oatmeal made with calcium-fortified soymilk with blueberries, sunflower seeds, and ground flaxseeds with calcium-fortified orange juice.

Snack: Figs, dates, raisins, and pecans.

Lunch: Grilled tempeh Reuben on a whole-grain bun served with coleslaw.

Snack: Granola, a banana, and soy yogurt.

Dinner: Soy cheese pizza with your choice of veggies and a small mixed-green salad.

Friday

Breakfast: Toaster waffles with a fruit salad of strawberries, bananas, and peaches and calcium-fortified orange juice.

Snack: Hummus with carrots and red pepper slices.

Lunch: Veggie chili with an avocado-tomato salad and baked corn chips.

Snack: Berry fruit smoothie made with vanilla soy yogurt and almonds.

Dinner: Lasagna with tofu, zucchini, and eggplant served with a small side salad and whole-grain garlic bread.

Saturday

Breakfast: Banana nut bread with soy butter and a fruit smoothie.

Snack: Granola bar and an apple and a glass of calcium-fortified orange juice.

Lunch: Minestrone soup and a small mixed-green salad.

Snack: Fruit salad sprinkled with wheat germ.

Dinner: Stuffed red bell pepper with ground soy meat, corn, scallions, tomatoes, and soy cheese and a side of brown rice.

Sunday

Breakfast: Flaxseed raisin bran with calcium-fortified rice milk and strawberries, soy bacon, and calcium-fortified orange juice.

Snack: Blueberry bran muffin with soy cream cheese and apple/carrot juice.

Lunch: Pita wrap with grilled zucchini, mushroom, eggplant, and hummus and a side of potato salad.

Snack: Fruit salad with raisins and almonds.

Dinner: Avocado roll, miso soup, and small salad with carrot ginger dressing.

BTW

- It's a given that all these foods should be organic whenever possible.

- Add a little organic flaxseed oil and blackstrap molasses to your fruit smoothies for extra omegas and iron.

- Make sure you're drinking tons of water!

- Our whore editor wants us to plug our cookbook, *Skinny Bitch in the Kitch*, here. So if you need help coming up with some new fun recipes, check it out. There are also a ton of other great veggie cookbooks out there. Google, bitches, google!

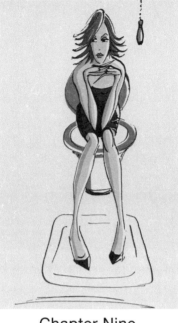

Chapter Nine
Pooping

L ay logs. Squeeze cheese. Take the Browns to the Superbowl. There are few things in life more satisfying than a well-crafted code brown. But pinching loaves isn't just for shits and giggles. Pooping is how we maintain a healthy weight, eliminate waste, and rid our bodies of toxins. Unfortunately, however, pregnancy can rob many of this simple pleasure.

Just so we're all on the same page—constipation is when you have trouble getting your poop out, you poop infrequently, or you only have really small, hard poops.[299] There are a few reasons constipation can flare up during pregnancy, some of which are beyond your control. For starters, pregnancy hormones can relax your intestinal muscles, slowing down the passage of food and waste.[300] Bummer. In addition, the baby can crowd your bowels, which makes your intestines narrower.[301] (Translation: Smaller poop chute.)

But don't go blaming your baby! Constipation can also be caused by a lot of other factors. So luckily, if you're causing your own misery, it can be easily remedied. If constipation was never an issue for you before, check with your doctor about your vitamins. Iron and calcium supplements can often be clogging culprits.[302] Sometimes switching brands, altering the dosage, or stopping altogether can make all the difference. (Obviously, you'll need to be meeting your iron and calcium needs through your diet. Check with your doctor.)[303]

And be sure you're drinking enough water every day. If you aren't, your cockadoodle-doo can become hard or dry, making pooping a real pain in the ass.

Are you sitting around all day like the Queen of Sheba? 'Cause that's not gonna help your cause. In fact, it increases the likelihood you'll be constipated.[304] Exercise not only gets your blood pumping, but it can also get your bowels brewing. Seriously. It makes a big difference in moving things along. You gotta move it to lose it!

Most important of all for anal action? Food, of course! Whatever you're putting in your mouth has a direct effect on what comes out your butt. So before you go blaming your vitamins or your growing fetus, check your diet, yo! All the while, bear in mind that fiber is important for your overall health, not just your arse: It can lower cholesterol, reduce risk of cancer, steady blood sugar, slow fat absorption, and curb overeating.[305] It's like a friggin' miracle! So which foods are high in fiber? At this point, it should come as no surprise: leafy greens, fresh fruit, whole wheat and other whole grains (in breads, muffins, cereals, and pastas), oats, barley, brown rice, potatoes, sweet potatoes, beans, legumes, raw or lightly steamed vegetables,[306] nuts, and seeds.[307] Eat a variety of these foods every day, and you'll be crapping like a champ in no time. (Just so you know, bananas are NOT binding.) And when you really need a stick of dynamite, dried figs (without added sugar or chemical preservatives), dates, prunes, and raspberries can do the trick.[308] Just be sure to drink plenty of water with your fiber. For fiber to work properly, there has to be an adequate amount of water in your body.[309]

Warning: If you're not used to eating high-fiber foods, be sure to ease in slowly. If you overload on fiber too quickly, you could have stomach pain, gas, bloating, or even a mudslide in your pants. But eventually, you do want to eat high-fiber foods all day, every day.

Which foods have little or no fiber? Again, it should come as no surprise: Meat, chicken, fish, eggs, milk, cheese, butter, and sugar.[310] Animal proteins are much harder for the body to digest than plant proteins (fruits, veggies, whole grains, nuts, seeds, legumes). Because the digestion process is slowed down during pregnancy, the last thing you want is undigested animal flesh putrefying in your stomach and intestines.[311] The resulting toxins aren't good for you or baby.[312] And neither are processed foods. Processed foods can have little to no fiber and are often pretty much worthless. Even "healthy" processed foods are less fibrous than their whole foods counterpart (i.e., apple sauce has less fiber than whole apples, orange juice has less fiber than whole oranges, etc.).

So when you're reaching for the potato chips instead of the baked potato, remember you're screwing yourself and your baby out of fiber. And unless you want gestational diabetes, reconsider your food choice. In a study of more than 13,000 women, it was found that higher intakes of good-quality fiber decreased the likelihood of gestational diabetes.[313]

If gestational diabetes doesn't scare you straight, maybe hemorrhoids will. You should be able to drop a deuce with ease; straining to lay cable can cause 'rroids![314] (Hemorrhoids are painful varicose veins in your cornhole! Arghhhhhh!) So get your shit together, or else!

But don't reach for the laxatives. Laxatives can rob your baby of both fluid and nutrients, and if used excessively, could possibly even lead to fetal abnormalities.[315] Stimulant laxatives can also cause contractions, which can lead to pre-term labor.[316] Eating fruits, veggies, legumes, and whole grains should stir up all the hiney heat you need.

Drink lots of water, eat well, and exercise, shitheads.

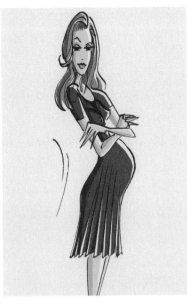

Chapter Ten
Trust No One

L et's face it: as Americans, we're the most spoiled people on the planet. We're fortunate enough to live in one of the most industrialized nations in the world—we have clean, running water and indoor plumbing; we dial 911 and real-life heroes show up on our doorsteps; and anything we could ever want comes in a hundred different shapes, sizes, and colors. Unfortunately, because we're so fortunate, we often take things for granted. We have our hands out all the time . . . "Gimme, gimme, gimme." And savvy entrepreneurs are all too happy to cash in on this mindset. Now granted, many companies sell products they believe in and are proud of. They actually care about being of service to consumers. But others are simply in it for the profit. It's estimated that there are 465,000 new businesses created every *month* in the United States![317] So how can you know which companies care and which companies don't? It's simple—you can't. So for your own safety and the safety of your unborn baby: Trust no one. While we like to think that most people are well intentioned and decent, a few bad apples can spoil the whole bunch.

Now, we don't need to tell you that our government is like one big company, do we? Yes, it's funded by our tax dollars, but make no mistake, it's still a business. And while the majority of our government employees may be honorable and good, there are certainly bad apples among them.

EPA

Take the Environmental Protection Agency (EPA), for example—a classic case of good guys vs. bad guys. In 2006, union leaders representing 9,000 EPA scientists and other employees filed a letter addressing EPA administrator Stephen

Johnson. They claimed that EPA managers and pesticide-industry officials were influencing scientists to skip steps when testing the safety of pesticides! Skip steps? Many of the pesticides in question stemmed from nerve gas research in World War II! Skip steps? It was reported that some pesticides could enter the brains of fetuses and young children and damage their developing nervous systems.[318] Skip @#$% steps? Pretty despicable, huh? You ain't seen nothin' yet. In August 2005 with bipartisan support, Congress enacted a moratorium—it mandated that the EPA stop testing toxic chemicals on humans until strict guidelines could be set. In addition, it required that the EPA draft a new rule permanently banning the testing of chemicals on pregnant women and children.[319] No ifs, ands, or buts. But the EPA instead proposed a rule filled with loopholes so unconscionable, it would make the devil himself blush:

- Children outside the United States would be fair game for chemical studies.
- Mentally impaired children as well as orphaned newborns could be studied, so long as there was permission from a parent, guardian, or care-taking institution.

- Children who were neglected or abused could be studied—
  no parental consent needed.[320]

Just so we're clear, studies all over the world have linked high pesticide levels in blood samples with cancer, birth defects, and neurological disorders.[321] And a recent study published in *Occupational and Environmental Medicine* revealed that children exposed to insecticides and pesticides have twice the risk for developing childhood leukemia. (Developing fetuses face the same statistics.)[322] So then why would the EPA want to study the effects of pesticides on children when we already know this? Hmm, does it have anything to do with the two million dollars they accepted from the American Chemistry Council (a group that represents insecticide manufacturers) for the CHEER study?[323] Shit if we know. But CHEERS (Children's Environmental Exposure Research Study) raised more eyebrows than Botox in Hollywood. The study was to take place in a low-income community, and in order to attract participants to the study, families were offered a free camcorder, $970, a bib, and a T-shirt. Uh-huh. In order to collect their booty, parents just needed to live in Duval County, Florida, and have a baby under three months old or between nine and twelve months old. Oh yeah, one more requirement according to the study's recruiting flyer: "spraying pesticides in your home routinely." Thankfully, Florida Senator Bill Nelson (and California Senator Barbara Boxer) threatened to block Stephen Johnson's confirmation if he allowed CHEERS to occur. The study was canceled.[324] (FYI: It was this whole debacle that preempted Congress to call for the aforementioned moratorium on human chemical testing.) Trust no one.

Did you have trouble getting pregnant? Researchers at Harvard, the University of Michigan, and the U.S. Centers for Disease Control did a study on men who had low sperm counts. They found that those with the lowest testosterone levels had the highest levels of chlorpyrifos in their urine.[325] Despite this frightening fact, chlorpyrifos is not only permissible for agricultural use, but according to the EPA, it's "one of the most widely used organophosphate insecticides."[326] Great, thanks.

Sadly, bullying scientists, poisoning children, and sterilizing men aren't the EPA's only missteps. Coal-fired power plants cause more uncontrolled mercury emissions than any other source.[327] The emissions rain down into bodies of water, get eaten or absorbed by fish, and then are ingested by people who eat the fish. (Everyone's susceptible to mercury's negative effects, but pregnant women, nursing mothers, fetuses, and small children are most at risk.)[328] In 2004, the EPA released an alarming study reporting that the blood tests of 630,000 newborns showed unsafe mercury levels. Yet just a few weeks after releasing the study, the EPA came up with a proposal that would make mercury matters even worse—allowing power plants to be exempt from installing pollution-reducing devices.[329] Eleven states opposed the EPA's proposal, asserting it was illegal under the Clean Air Act and would pose a health risk to citizens.[330]

In the EPA's defense, in 2003, they aimed to reduce mercury emissions 90 percent by 2008. But for reasons unjustifiable to the rest of the free world, the Bush administration suggested 70 percent by 2018. If that's not horrifying enough, it was also proposed that mercury be de-listed as a toxic air pollutant![331] Why would anyone on the planet want to allow such catastrophic pollution to continue? Um, maybe because it's really lucrative? Republican election campaigns received $40 million from the energy industry; George W. Bush alone received $1.3 million.[332] Trust no one.

USDA

Tsk, tsk, George W. Bush. Tsk, tsk. But your friends at the USDA aren't much better. According to the watchdog group Organic Consumers Association, "Lester Friedlander, a former USDA veterinarian, says he was told by USDA officials as far back as 1991 that if his testing ever found evidence of mad cow disease, he was to tell no one. He and other scientists say they know of cases where cows tested positive for the disease in laboratories but were ruled negative by the USDA."[333] Maybe that's why the USDA currently tests less than one-tenth of one percent of cows for mad cow disease.

When a Kansas-based meatpacking company decided to test all its animals for the disease, the USDA threatened to prosecute.[334] Huh? It wasn't going to cost the USDA a dime—it would be done at the company's own expense. And the primary function of the USDA is to keep our food safe. So why in the hell would they want to stop a meatpacking company from testing its animals for mad cow disease? Well, for starters, many high-ranking officials at the USDA have direct ties with the meat and dairy industries—the industries they're supposed to be protecting us from! The USDA Agriculture Secretary from January 2001 until January 2005 not only had ties with Monsanto, the company responsible for producing the controversial bovine growth hormone (BGH), but she was also linked to a major meatpacking corporation.[335]

The buck doesn't stop there. She employed a spokeswoman who was the former public relations director for the National Cattlemen's Beef Association, a chief of staff who used to be its head lobbyist, a former president of the National Pork Producers Council, and former executives from the meatpacking industry, to name a few![336] Um, hello? Conflict of interest! No wonder staffers at the USDA fought against private testing for mad cow disease—they didn't want to anger their buddies in the meatpacking industry. Or, according to one watchdog group, "The USDA obviously doesn't want the private sector to start testing for mad cow disease in the USA, because they know the disease is here, and it is spreading."[337] That's possible. Or, perhaps they know if private meatpacking companies start testing all their animals, no one will want to buy USDA meat anymore. Translation: "If other companies start testing, our farmers have to start testing. And that's going to cost money." Either way, it's downright sinister. Thankfully, the judge ruled in favor of the meatpacking company.[338]

But judges aren't always around. In 1990, Congress passed

legislation to create the National Organic Standards Board (NOSB), a group that would develop and oversee organic standards. In order to create a balanced Board, federal law mandated that it must be comprised of four farmers, three environmentalists, three consumer advocates, two handlers/processors, one certifying agent, one retailer, and one scientist. Great. All fair. But in 2005, the USDA handed over a *consumer advocate seat* to a consultant for the dairy industry,[339] a *scientist* seat went to a manager at General Mills, an *environmentalist* seat to was given to a representative from a mushroom farm, and *a consumer and public interest* seat was handed off to a representative from a primarily non-organic farm![340] It's like asking a pride of lions to keep an eye on your baby!

That's not the first time the USDA has messed with organics, and surely it won't be the last. In 2006, they sought to allow more synthetic chemicals into "organic" meat. Livestock could be treated with an anti-diarrhea drug, a pre-surgical painkiller, an anti-inflammatory, a diuretic, a synthetic stool softener, and a sanitizing disinfectant,[341] just to name a few. Does that sound like organic meat to you? As recently as 2007, the USDA approved an interim rule to allow thirty-eight *non-organic* ingredients to be used in *organic* products!

So you'd be a buying a product that says "USDA Organic," on the label, but really, it's not![342] If you're not absolutely appalled, you're not paying attention. Put the book down and go take a nap. It is essential that we have at least *one* safe food source, and organics is all we've got. If the USDA robs us of this by allowing industry to trample organic standards, we're screwed.

It's bad enough they barely appropriate any funds for organics, one of the largest growing food sectors. In 2006, of the USDA's $90 billion annual budget, a measly $5 million was allocated for organic farming research! The National Organic Program, which is in charge of regulating the entire industry in the United States, has only nine employees![343]

Now, you may be thinking, "Who cares about organic? Only rich snobs can afford it, anyway." If that's the case, *you're* being a snob, and you need to get with the program. Pesticide exposure has been linked to learning disabilities, behavioral disorders, developmental delays, and dysfunctional motor skills. Yet, at this time, more than *300* synthetic chemicals can be used regularly in conventional farming. Conversely, *none* are allowed in organic farming. According to the U.S. Centers for Disease Control, one of the main sources of pesticide exposure for kids is food. Blood samples revealed pesticide concentrations six times higher in children who ate conventional produce compared with kids who ate organic. Laboratory tests found sixteen different pesticides in eight top-selling baby foods—three of which were carcinogenic![344] Eating food free of chemical pesticides is a God-given right; it shouldn't just be for the privileged. And if our United States Department of Agriculture agreed with this notion, they'd do everything in their power to make it readily available to *everyone*. Trust no one.

FDA

As part of its mission statement, the Food and Drug Administration—the FDA—claims responsibility for the "safety . . . and security . . . of our nation's food supply . . ."[345] Really? That's strange, because they allow more than three friggin' hundred synthetic food chemicals into conventionally produced foods![346] We don't know what's worse—that or their announcement on December 29, 2006, that meat and milk from cloned animals are safe for human consumption. Yeah, despite the fact that as many as 99 percent of these poor Franken-animals have heart, brain, liver, and kidney disorders;

skeletal malformations; genetic abnormalities; and an exorbitantly high fetal death rate, the FDA says their meat and milk are just as "safe" as regular animals'. As of publication time, the decision to allow these products on the shelves isn't final. But if upheld, because the almighty FDA deemed them "safe," the law won't require any labels notifying consumers that they're buying cloned products.[347] Their sick, twisted reasoning for this: It just wouldn't be fair to the farmers of cloned animals. If these foods are just as "safe," but consumers have a negative association with them, they won't get purchased. Better to hide the truth and take away consumers' rights to decide for themselves.

We shouldn't be surprised the organization, as a whole, is so unscrupulous. When the nonprofit group Union of Concerned Scientists sent a survey to nearly 6,000 FDA scientists, only about 1,000 responded. Why such a small amount? Of those who did respond, 40 percent feared "retaliation for voicing safety concerns in public." Equally alarming, more than 33 percent "did not feel they could express safety concerns even inside the agency." Doubly alarming: Almost 20 percent said that they "have been asked, for non-scientific reasons, to inappropriately exclude or alter technical information or their conclusions in an FDA scientific document." Alarming and tragic: Only 47 percent think the "FDA routinely provides complete and accurate information to the public."[348]

DON'T GET MAD, GET ACTIVE!

If you feel like running away and living on Mars, we don't blame you. It's stuff like this that compelled us to write books. Get mad, but only for a minute (it's not good for the baby). Then, get active. Go to www.congress.org to get contact information for senators, representatives, the president, and vice president and demand the reform of these crooked, self-serving agencies. And until hell freezes over, trust no one!

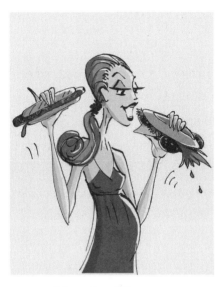

Chapter Eleven
Cravings: The Monster Inside

"*I have to* have something sweet after every meal." "I would die without cheese." "I'm craving meat; I must need iron." Oh puh-lease. Save the drama for your mama. Say hello to your cravings—dark, evil, compulsive thoughts hell-bent on running your life. People always assume that their cravings are reliable indicators of what their bodies need... until they acknowledge that cigarette smokers crave cigarettes, drug addicts crave drugs, and alcoholics crave alcohol. In that sense, your body does need what it craves. When you do something harmful to your body, your body's army fights back. Imagine these little soldiers suiting up for battle, ready to go to war. But when you suddenly stop giving your body the harmful substance, the soldiers are still present, raring to go. It's the presence of these soldiers—without anything to attack—that are your cravings.

If it's dairy you're craving, it might actually be a drug addiction! Cows' milk has traces of morphine in it! Morphine, along with codeine and other opiates, are naturally produced in cows' livers and end up in their milk.[349] But that's not all. All milk, whether from a cow or a human, contains casein, a protein that breaks apart during digestion and releases a whole slew of opiates. All these "feel good" chemicals exist so that newborns will nurse and thrive and to ensure a bond between mothers and their young.[350] When a woman breastfeeds, her milk has an almost drug-like effect on the baby. The baby is totally hooked. He'll cry, not because he's hungry, but because he needs a "fix" of that pleasurable feeling produced by the opiates. Mother Nature has guaranteed that our babies will nurse and grow. And she's done the same for all mammals. We slowly wean our offspring from our milk, the addiction is gently broken, and all is well. But after we "get off" our own casein, we humans start ingesting the casein of other animals. All dairy products contain casein, but cheese has the highest concentration. In fact, cheese contains far more casein than is naturally found in cows' milk. It also has phenylethylamine, an amphetamine-like chemical. So when we kid around and say, "I am addicted to cheese," it's not a joke—it's true. We are chemically addicted to cheese.[351] The following hormones and natural chemicals have all been identified in cows' milk: prolactin, somatostatin, melatonin, oxytocin, growth hormone, leuteinizing-releasing hormone, thyrotropin-releasing hormone, thyroid-stimulating hormone, vasoactive intestinal peptide, calcitonin, parathyroid hormone, corticos-teroids, estrogens, progesterone, insulin, epidermal growth factor, insulin-like growth factor, erythropoietin, bombesin, neurotensin, motilin, and cholecystokinin.[352] If you think your will is strong enough to conquer all those mother#$@%s, you're on drugs!

So assuming you're not smoking, drinking, or doing dairy drugs, why are you having these crazy-ass food cravings? Well, there are about as many theories for cravings as there are for morning sickness. One theory points to food addiction in relation to food intolerance. Meaning, as strange as it sounds, we could be drawn to the very foods that our bodies are most sensitive to. For example, someone completely obsessed with cheese or ice cream could actually be lactose intolerant. While this sounds totally off the wall, it does make sense when you look at cigs and booze and drugs—people who are hooked on them can't get enough, despite how harmful they are.[353] Now again, this is just one theory. So please don't get all neurotic and think that if you're craving bananas, you must be allergic to them. Especially since some experts think cravings might just be psychological.[354] Like, if your whole life you hear that pregnant women crave pickles and ice cream, when you get pregnant, you may be preprogrammed to crave pickles and ice cream. If your cravings aren't psychological, they may be emotional. Some women approach pregnancy-eating with a sense of entitlement: "I've been starving myself to be thin all these years so now I'm gonna eat whatever I want." Others get nostalgic for their favorite childhood treats or foods that remind them of their religious or cultural backgrounds.[355]

However, most researchers agree that there's no hard, scientific proof for what causes cravings.[356] But interestingly enough, some cravings may indicate the body needs something.

Now, maybe the pickle and olives thing was preprogrammed. But it's also possible that your body wants more sodium. Progesterone causes the body to excrete sodium at an increased rate. And because blood volume increases, the intake of more sodium is necessary to maintain a healthy balance.[357] (But don't get your sodium from canned, processed junk. Just use sea salt to season your food to taste.)

Totally fascinating: Pica, a condition observed throughout the world, has pregnant women craving—get this—clay. Apparently, clay is a natural digestive aid and can help combat toxins and nausea. In Zambia, some pregnant women take a clay medicine for stomach upset. However, because it is typically laden with lead and other harmful elements, Western medicine typically advises pregnant women to avoid eating clay.[358] Also lumped into the "pica" category is the desire to eat dirt, baking soda, laundry starch, toilet paper, chalk,[359] and even cigarette butts![360] Now, none of these items are renowned for high iron content, but it's been reported that women craving these items may be deficient in iron.[361] None of these cravings have been scientifically proven to translate to iron deficiency. However, the craving for ice, of all things, has been well documented and may be an indicator of anemia.[362]

So be on the lookout. And while you're at it, keep your eyes on your chocolate addiction. Again, not scientifically proven, but for what it's worth, some alternative medicine practitioners feel that chocolate cravings may signify a shortage of B vitamins.[363]

So what do you do when the cravings creep up? Well, for starters, know that you're not alone. One study found that 61 percent of pregnant women experienced food cravings.[364] Another reported as many as 80 percent.[365] Don't let the pull of the dark side draw you in. You are the force, Luke. But if Jedi mind-tricks won't keep your cravings at bay, following some simple advice will. First and foremost, always be prepared. Have healthy food on hand at all times. It's amazing how hunger can make people crazy—especially pregnant people. Don't think that you can get through a day without eating crap on sheer willpower. You can't. If you're hungry, and you don't have something healthy on hand, you will definitely eat whatever shit is most accessible.

Be sure to eat breakfast every single day. If you don't, you may experience even worse cravings than usual.[366] The best defense against cravings is a good offense—head them off before they can rear their ugly heads. Because once they kick in, your resolve will likely be totally weakened. Especially if you're craving something sweet. Even though we often associate a sugar urge with a lack of self-control, it can frequently just be a case of hypoglycemia (low blood sugar). The craving is simply the body's way of trying to replenish sugar quickly.[367] So don't let it come to that. Stabilize, bitches. Stabilize.

And be sure you aren't mistaking a necessary carb fueling for a sugar craving. In that case, eating fruit, a sweet potato, a muffin, bagel, pasta, or piece of bread made from whole grains will do the trick.[368] If you're all set with carbs and actually *are* having a sweet craving, believe it or not, you can avoid a sugarfest by eating fruit, drinking peppermint tea, or brushing your teeth.

A trick for fighting cravings in general is drinking two glasses of water and waiting fifteen minutes. What was presenting as a wicked case of the munchies can be easily and healthily remedied by hydration.[369] If that doesn't seem to help, try some flaxseed oil. (Add it to your salad or in your fruit smoothies.) One midwife and herbalist theorized that her patients' cravings were caused by a deficit in essential fatty acids. She found that when they took flaxseed oil, their cravings vanished.[370]

Lastly, and most important, eat, eat, eat. Load up on healthy meals. This way, snack attacks will be just that, and not actual hunger. Don't confuse the two. If you don't address hunger, you'll be gorging on junk, instead of occasionally indulging in it.

Yeah, we said, "indulging." According to a national survey, 75 percent of cravers admitted to partaking in crap, while only 8 percent sought a healthy alternative.[371] While we'd love nothing more than for you to be one of the 8 percent, statistically, it's unlikely. So know that if you do eat shit occasionally in small doses, it's not the end of the world—you're not gonna give birth to a goat or something. The only thing worse than a pregnant woman eating junk is a pregnant woman eating junk and then worrying about it. What good does worrying do? It doesn't serve you or your baby at all. In fact, it's bad for both of you. So do the best you can, be imperfect, and be okay with it. Just try not to eat crap on an empty stomach. Eating something unhealthy alongside something healthy can be less jarring on the body.[372] So if you insist on eating a box of cookies, eat some steamed broccoli and brown rice first. (Just kidding about the "box" of cookies. Don't you dare eat a whole box!)

Now for some of you, just the thought of broccoli may make you want to puke. Food aversions during pregnancy are as common as cravings. So what do you do if healthy foods hold no appeal? First off, use your head. If oranges gross you out, choose another food high in vitamin C, like tomatoes or kiwis. If green leafy veggies revolt you, get your beta-carotene fix from peaches or apricots.[373] Work around your aversions and just do the best you can. It's more important to feel good about your food choices than obsess about them.

And if you do give birth to a baby goat, surely you'll love him anyway.

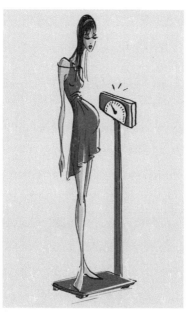

Chapter Twelve
Skinny Mama?

Part of the reason we chose this book's title is because we have wildly inappropriate senses of humor. But the main reason is because we knew it would get the attention of all you vain-ass broads. We totally get the irony of suggesting a pregnant woman should be skinny. There are few things more ridiculous. You have a baby growing and developing inside your body. Now is not the time to be concerned about your figure! If you allow your vanity to affect your pregnancy, you're asking for serious trouble. Women who don't gain enough weight are more likely to give birth prematurely,[374] and they increase their risk of having a baby with low birth weight (LBW). LBW babies are more likely to suffer from asthma, ear infections, and respiratory tract infections. In addition, they're more likely to have childhood psychological disorders, developmental delays, and lower intelligence test scores.[375] If you bought this book because you actually thought you'd find a way to stay skinny throughout your pregnancy or you're otherwise struggling with the weight-gain issue, please, please, please talk to your doctor or midwife. Together, you can address your concerns and make sure you don't put your baby's health at risk. So how much weight should you gain? That all depends on your pre-pregnancy weight:

If you were underweight before, you should gain 28–40 pounds total. Depending on how underweight you were and what your doctor recommends, you should gain about 5–6 pounds (or more) in the first trimester and about 1–2 pounds per week in the second and third trimesters.

If you were a healthy weight before, you should gain 25–35 pounds total. You should gain about 3–5 pounds in the first trimester and about 1–2 pounds per week in the second and third trimesters.

According to the vast majority of sources, if you were overweight before, you should gain 15–25 pounds total—about 1–2 pounds in the first trimester and about 1 pound per week in the second and third trimesters.[376] Even in the case of obesity, almost every source says pregnant women should gain this weight and should not lose any. However, a new study published in the June 2007 issue of *Journal of Applied Physiology, Nutrition, and Metabolism* had interesting results. The study included ninety-six obese pregnant women with gestational diabetes (also known as gestational diabetes mellitus, or GDM). It was found that, "caloric restriction and exercise result in limited weight gain in obese subjects with GDM, less macrosomic neonates [babies large for gestational age—in a bad way], and no adverse pregnancy outcomes." Translation: Obese pregnant women with gestational diabetes who *didn't* gain weight didn't suffer any adverse complications with their pregnancies or babies and were less likely to have large babies. So according to this study, if you're obese and suffering from gestational diabetes, it may be okay not to gain any weight during your pregnancy.[377] Now, it's just one study, it contradicts popular opinion, and they only had ninety-six subjects. So if you are obese, discuss this study with your doctor, and together decide what you should do. Whatever you do, don't worry: Most women who are overweight still have healthy pregnancies and deliver without complications.[378]

If you've got two buns in the oven—twins—you should gain about 35–45 pounds. But weight gain for multiple births should be carefully monitored by your doctor.[379]

While these are the ideals, don't be alarmed if you don't fit them exactly. Some women have such bad morning sickness in the first trimester, they actually lose a little weight. So while you do want to gain weight steadily throughout your pregnancy, it's okay if you lose a little weight in the beginning. Mother Nature, in all her infinite wisdom, made it so that babies don't require as many calories and nutrients in the first trimester as they do later on.[380] (For all you psychos obsessed with being thin: This does NOT mean you should avoid gaining weight early on in your pregnancy.) Just be sure to keep your healthcare provider apprised of your situation.

It's totally understandable to be weirded out by all the changes occurring in your body. So knowing how all the weight gets distributed may make you feel a little better. It's actually kinda cool:

• Baby: 6–8 pounds

- Placenta: 1–2 pounds
- Fluids in maternal tissue: 2–4 pounds
- Uterus: 2 pounds
- Boobs: 1–2 pounds
- Blood volume: 3–4 pounds
- Amniotic fluid: 2 pounds
- Fat and nutrient stores: 4–7 pounds[381]

See? You're not a buffalo. You've got all sorts of extra blood and guts and fluids weighing you down, all of which are necessary. (Plus you get boobs!) So get over the weight gain.

But don't go hog wild. Gaining too much weight can bring on a whole slew of problems: back pain, leg pain, varicose veins, fatigue, high blood pressure, gestational diabetes, and an increased chance of needing a C-section.[382] But you're not the only one who'll suffer. Gaining too much pregnancy weight can have serious consequences for your baby, too. According to a recent Harvard study, our kids are as affected by the obesity epidemic as the rest of us. Children six years and under are 59 percent more likely to be overweight than they were twenty years ago. Babies six months and under are 74 percent more likely.[383] According to Emily Oken, MD,

MPH, and lead author of another Harvard study, "excessive weight gain during pregnancy [is] directly associated with having an overweight child. Just like adults, children who are overweight are at a higher risk for a number of health conditions such as high blood pressure, diabetes, and high cholesterol."[384] Through no fault of their own, children are starting their lives with one big strike against them. Make that two strikes: Babies born to obese moms are almost twice as likely to be premature or have birth defects.[385] Actually, it's three strikes: Another study under way suggests that overweight children may be at a higher risk for asthma.[386]

We aren't trying to scare, shame, or upset you. We really aren't. We want this to be the most wonderful, happy time in your life, and we don't want you worrying or obsessing about anything. But at the same time, we want you to know the truth. (So don't be sending hate mail our way, like, we're making you feel bad for telling you what science says.) Your baby's life literally depends on you making healthy, informed choices about what you eat. If you already are overweight, do not worry yourself sick! We had to include this information so other women wouldn't eat recklessly throughout their pregnancies. But you're going to be fine, and so is your baby.

Plenty of women are obese these days and delivering perfectly fine, perfectly beautiful babies. So if you've spent your whole life being plagued by bad eating habits, don't despair. Get excited to finally turn things around. From today on, start making healthier choices—for you and your baby!

That includes exercising, girls. Just because you're a waddling weeble-wobble doesn't mean you get to sit around all day, sedentary. In fact, according to the American College of Obstetricians and Gynecologists, pregnant women (without any health issues) should aim to exercise moderately for thirty minutes or more on most, if not all, days of the week. You heard us. Unless you have a pass from your doctor, move your fat ass every day for thirty minutes! But if you've been lying around on the couch for the last twenty years, ease in slowly. And be smart about what type of exercise you choose. Clearly, football, soccer, softball, horseback riding, gymnastics, kickboxing, downhill skiing, hockey, and the like should be avoided. Use your head—nothing that'll hit your stomach, shake the baby, or risk injury or falling. And no exercising in altitudes above 6,000 feet or scuba diving at all.[387]

Exercise can be invaluable in making your pregnancy healthy and happy. For starters, it can help with constipation, backaches, fatigue, and varicose veins. And not only can it aid in improving your sleep, but it also reduces the risk of high blood pressure, diabetes, depression, and anxiety.[388] Hello? Who wouldn't want all that! Not sold? How about this: Active women have shorter labors, easier deliveries, quicker recovery times, and can get back into shape faster postpartum.[389] And of course, what's good for mom is good for baby. Exercise gets the blood circulating, which positively affects the placenta (which gives the baby oxygen and nutrients).[390]

So get to steppin'. But whether you were a gym rat prior or this will be your first time ever, check with your doctor or midwife before getting started. Exercise may not be safe if you have any of the following issues: more than one bun in the oven, risk of premature labor, heart or lung disease, bleeding, preeclampsia, placenta previa, ruptured membranes,[391] complications with past pregnancies, thyroid disease, severe diabetes, seizure disorders,[392] asthma, anemia, muscle or joint problems, repeated C-sections, previous miscarriage, a sedentary lifestyle, or you're extremely over- or underweight.[393]

Assuming you get the green light from your healthcare provider, be sure you always drink tons of water before, during, and after exercise. And be extra careful. You've got a big belly, big boobs, and you aren't as graceful as you were before. It's really easy to fall doing simple stuff—like walking. So even if you feel lithe and agile, proceed with caution. Especially when stretching. All your ligaments and joints are looser than ever, allowing your body to expand for baby. Overstretching will not do you any good. And neither will lying flat on your back. After sixteen weeks (your fourth month of pregnancy), avoid doing any exercise that has you in that position. The weight of your newly heavy uterus on a major blood vessel can affect blood flow to the placenta.[394]

Sounds like a good excuse to avoid having sex, huh? Sorry, no such luck. Sex is great exercise, so just get on top. But whether you're having sex or exercising, if you experience any of the following, stop immediately and call your doctor: dizziness, blurred vision, chest pains, headaches, vaginal leaking or bleeding, contractions, abdominal pain, or calf swelling or pain.[395] On the other hand, if you experience multiple orgasms, thank your lucky stars, then your husband/partner, and call everyone you know to brag about it.

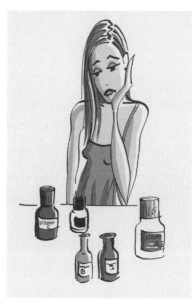

Chapter Thirteen

Stupid, Boring Vitamin Chapter

Okay, so maybe you've figured it out by now. If you haven't, let us spell it out for you: Your baby is like a parasite growing inside you. And you are the host body. So whether your little parasite thrives or not is entirely up to you. (Charming, huh?) We cannot emphasize enough the importance of having a healthy host body for your baby. For starters, your baby's life depends on it, literally. But it also means the difference between you glowing or growling for nine months.

So in addition to resting often, exercising regularly, and giving up junk food, you need to be sure you're getting all your vitamins and minerals. The best way to do this: Eat a variety of healthy foods. Our bodies absorb vitamins and minerals from food better than they do from supplements, and good food supplies thousands of protective components you won't find in a pill. So even though your healthcare provider will likely have you popping pills on a daily basis, there's no substitute for healthy eating. At this point in the book, we've probably said it a thousand times, but we're saying it again: Eat a well-balanced diet of fruits, veggies, whole grains, nuts, seeds, and legumes. And be sure to change it up so you aren't eating the same exact foods every day for nine months. This will ensure you're getting a good variety of vitamins and minerals and nutrients.

And don't be a cheap jerk. Buy organic! Studies show that conventional produce has significantly less phosphorous, iron, calcium, protein, riboflavin, and ascorbic acid than it did fifty years ago. Why? Because of all the chemical fertilizers, pesticides, and monoculture farming practices that came with the industrialization of our food production. Fortunately, studies show that organic produce has higher levels of vitamins, minerals, and antioxidants.[396] Do not shrug this off. Vitamins, minerals, and antioxidants are everything to your health and your baby's health. Pesticides can cross the placenta and cause neurological and reproductive damage to your unborn baby. Get in the habit now, because when your *baby* is a *child*, he or she will still need you to buy organic food. In 2003, a report from the Centers for Disease Control & Prevention found the urine of children tested *twice* as high as the urine of adults for some pesticides. And let's not forget the University of Washington study on preschoolers. Those fed conventional diets tested *six times* higher for certain pesticides than the kids fortunate enough to be fed organic diets.[397] So decide right now what kind of mom you want to be. Loving or lacking.

According to some research, the diets of pregnant women may be lacking in folic acid, calcium, magnesium, iron, zinc, and vitamins B-6, D, and E.[398] But like everything else in the world of health, there's a lot of conflicting information out there. Especially regarding vitamin supplements. Some researchers say, "Better safe than sorry," and advise pregnant women to take a multi-vitamin. Others suggest just taking supplements for the things you could be deficient in. And some even say there's no reason to supplement at all if you're eating a well-planned, well-balanced diet and all your levels are good. So we're gonna present you with a broad overview of what we've learned and let you decide, with the help of your healthcare provider, what's best for you. Remember: We're not the end-all, be-all on anything. So don't be writing to us, asking, "What should I do about vitamins?" Ask your doctor for the most current RDAs on vitamins and minerals, read more on the subject from other sources, and then make an educated decision with his or her help. And be sure you develop a game plan regarding supplementation for pregnancy and breastfeeding.

(Warning: There's nothing more boring than talking about vitamins. Sorry in advance.)

While there is a ton of conflicting information, one thing experts do agree on is that alcohol, tobacco, soda, sugar, and highly processed junk foods can cause the body to excrete vital vitamins and minerals. Another area of agreement is the importance of folic acid. Hopefully, you were taking it before you got preggers. (If you weren't, don't start freaking out now.) But it's also important during your first trimester, as deficiencies can cause neural tube defects. You can get it from fruits, veggies, whole grains, nuts, seeds, and legumes (of course).[399] But most experts say, in addition to the folic acid you're getting from your food, you should also take 400 micrograms a day.[400]

Your doctor may suggest taking a supplement that has all the B vitamins. You can give your body extra help by eating a variety of fruits, veggies, leafy greens, whole grains, legumes, nuts, and seeds. However, in the case of veggies (and fruits, too), cooking or overcooking can cause a loss of vitamins (and flavor too). So if you can't eat them raw, try lightly steaming them. And if you have to boil them, just do it for the minimum time possible. They should still look alive, crisp, and brightly colored when you're done cooking them. They shouldn't look lifeless, mushy, or dull.[401] Also be aware that high intakes of sugar, coffee, alcohol, nicotine, and black tea can cause nutrient depletion.[402]

If you've decided to eliminate meat, eggs and dairy products from your diet, feel good about it. And know that plant foods contain all the vitamins except vitamins D and B-12. (We don't say this meaning you should ignore your doctor's orders for supplements. We just thought you'd like to know that, in general, plant foods have all the vitamins except D and B-12.) You may remember from earlier on that you can get vitamin D from sun exposure on your skin (though if you live in a northern climate this will be harder to do). And of course you can eat D-fortified foods like cereal and rice- or soy-milks. And while small amounts of vitamin B-12 are present in bacteria, algae, tempeh, and fortified foods, vegetarian mothers-to-be should take supplements.[403] (FYI: Many experts say *all* vegetarians should take B-12 supplements, not just pregnant women.)

So be sure to discuss B-12 supplementation with your doctor, for both pregnancy and breastfeeding. It's a really important one for you and your baby. Babies born to moms who are deficient in B-12 can have anemia, developmental delays, impaired growth, and poor brain development.[404]

Believe it or not, vegetarians and vegans eating a well-balanced, well-planned diet can have better levels of most vitamins and minerals than meat-eaters. You may wonder about iron. While our levels can be lower than average, they're still in the normal range. So when some meathead tells you that vegetarians or vegans don't get enough iron, tell him or her that we have no higher incidence of iron deficiency anemia than the general population. [405] Regardless, do your best to eat iron-rich foods, like almonds, asparagus, avocados, chickpeas, black beans, lentils, apricots, prunes, wheat germ, whole-wheat bread, sesame seeds, white beans, cherries, broccoli, leafy greens, beets, carrots, fortified cereals, and rice- and soymilks. You can help your body optimize iron absorption by pairing up high-iron foods with high vitamin-C foods. Your doctor may test your iron levels throughout your pregnancy to make sure you aren't anemic. If you are, you might have to take iron supplements, which can cause nausea, barfing, stomach upset, or constipation. (It can also inhibit zinc absorption.)[406] So eat right, fool!

Vitamin A is another one you gotta watch out for. While it is important for the fetus' cells and organs, too much vitamin A from animal sources (also known as retinol) can increase the chances of birth defects. So make sure you're not getting more than 10,000 international units (IU) of vitamin A per day. The good news is that no risk is associated with beta-carotene, the vitamin A that comes from plants.[407] Vitamin A abounds in all yellow and orange fruits and veggies, like mangos, apricots, peaches, papayas, carrots, squash, pumpkin, yams, and sweet potatoes. Hell, it's even in some non-yellow and -orange foods, like cherries, seaweeds, spinach, and broccoli.[408] Let's hear it for plants, yo!

Especially 'cause they're great for calcium, too! (You

should remember this from the dairy chapter, but we'll go ahead and refresh your memory.) Calcium is naturally abundant in and readily absorbed from many leafy greens (kale, mustard greens, collard greens, turnip greens), bok choy, cabbage, broccoli, Brussels sprouts, okra, watercress, chickpeas, red beans, soybeans, almonds, sesame seeds, and sea vegetables (like seaweed). It can also be attained from fortified orange juice, soymilk, rice milk, cereal, and calcium-processed tofu. So now you know how to get calcium, but how can you help your body keep it around? Regular exercise! Yep, it's true! Also, getting enough vitamin D and other nutrients (like vitamin K and magnesium) helps your body get the most out of calcium. [409]

Phosphorous is another winner. It's important for tissue repair, muscle contraction, production of RNA and DNA, maintenance of teeth and bones, and conversion of fats and carbs into energy. You can get good amounts of phosphorous from nuts, seeds, tofu, and whole grains. [410]

And you can get zinc, an important mineral, from tofu, legumes, beets, peanuts, Brazil nuts, and pumpkin seeds (the best source). [411] Zinc is critical to develop the thymus, [412] help carry to term, ensure a good birth weight, and promote adequate growth. A severe deficiency can cause serious problems.[413]

Actually, many minerals are important, but we'll all die of boredom if we go over every single one. So we're just gonna touch on selenium, iodine, copper, manganese, and magnesium.[414] Selenium, an antioxidant good for the immune system, can be obtained from Brazil nuts (the best source), brown rice, sunflower seeds, and tofu.[415] Iodine, necessary for thyroid function and cell oxygenation,[416] can be found in seaweed, kelp, and sea salt. (You can also get iodine from iodized salt, but you can easily go overboard. Too much can cause iodine toxicity, which suppresses thyroid function.)[417] Copper, important for the development of your baby's brain and immune system, can be found in nuts and beans. And nuts, seeds, and grains are good sources of manganese, which prevents birth defects.[418] You can get magnesium from leafy greens, whole grains, sea veggies, and nuts, but the highest concentrations are in sesame, sunflower, and pumpkin seeds. Oh, and dark chocolate, too. (Settle down.) Magnesium is a real over-achiever, contributing to more than three hundred different biological functions. But what you'll be most interested to learn: A study of women in West Germany found that those who took 400 milligrams of magnesium daily had fewer miscarriages and fewer pregnancy complications. Magnesium also plays a supporting role in making DHA.[419]

DHA is a fatty acid, and it's vital for brain development and visual acuity in infants. While DHA supplementing hasn't been popular long (compared to the other viteys), it's paramount that pregnant and nursing moms get adequate supplies. Otherwise, in addition to insufficient brain and vision development, your child may also be at a higher risk for ADD, OCD, and depression.[420] And it's been suggested that low DHA levels can cause depression and postpartum depression in moms.[421] While you can get DHA from eating fish, you'd also be getting all the contaminants and toxic pollutants that were absorbed into the fish's flesh. So instead, you can get your DHA from the same source the fish gets it—microalgae, tiny sea plants. Luckily, you don't have to go trolling the ocean floor; DHA microalgae supplements are available. If you can't find them in your local health store, get 'em online at Vegetarianvitamin.com (Deva Vegan Omega-3 DHA softgels) or Veganessentials.com (Udo's DHA Oil Blend or O-mega-Zen3 Liquid Vegan DHA Supplement by NuTru). As usual, consult your doctor. But be sure he or she knows about the DHA study that found fewer than 2 percent of pregnant or lactating woman to have adequate DHA levels.[122] And of course, avoid alcohol, smoking, saturated fats, trans fatty acids, white sugar, high dietary cholesterol intake, being malnourished, or taking unnecessary medication. All these, in addition to obesity, can cause problems with DHA production or conversion.[423]

By the way, DHA is one of the omega-3 fatty acids, along with its sister EPA. The body can make them from ALA (the mama omega-3), but it's a great idea to get DHA and EPA where you can. This is important, so pay attention: We generally get enough, and likely too much omega-6, because according to some experts, the ratio of omega-6 to omega-3s shouldn't be so high. So in order to improve the ratio and be sure you're getting enough omega-3s, include omega-3-rich foods every day. Flax seed oil is particularly high in omega 3s, but you can overdo it, which is potentially damaging. So if you use flaxseed oil, have no more than two teaspoons per day. Also, take one DHA/EPA capsule a day (providing about 0.3 grams of readily available omega-3s) as an insurance policy.[424] Walnuts, walnut oil, canola oil, and some green leafy veggies are all sources of ALA. ALA is converted in the body into EPA (and to a lesser extent, DHA, too).[425] They're all important for all pregnant women, but especially those who are vegan. So talk to your doctor about these omega-3s and make sure you're up to snuff. There are other important essential fatty acids, too. GLA is also one that, if you have a low level of it, you may be more prone to depression. It's another you'll want to talk about with your doctor and consider supplementing.

Whatever you do, don't let fatty acids get you all worked up. If you do, you may need to load up on everyone's favorite: vitamin C. During stressful times, the body uses more vitamin C than usual. So if you're feeling a little frazzled, load up on vitamin C–rich foods (or check with your doctor about supplementing). Vitamin C can be found in almost every fruit and vegetable, but notably berries, melons, citrus fruits, tomatoes, kiwis, mangos, green veggies (Brussels sprouts, spinach, collard greens, broccoli, asparagus, peppers, cabbage), and potatoes. It's vital for immune system function, connective tissue formation, hormone production, and protection from free-radical buildup.[426]

Vitamin E, too, offers protection from free radicals, but it's also vital for optimal nervous and immune system function,[427] development of the pituitary gland,[428] and helping you and your baby use oxygen most efficiently. Vitamin E can be found in nuts, seeds, their oils, vegetable oils, and whole grains. Talk to your doctor to see if supplementing is right for you, especially since vitamin E has been known to prevent miscarriage.[429]

While all vitamins and minerals are important during pregnancy and breastfeeding, the ones you should pay special attention to (especially if you're vegetarian or vegan) are: B-12, vitamin D, and EFAs (essential fatty acids). Talk to your doctor!

(Nerd alert: If you want extra credit, do a little research on chlorella, spirulina, and nutritional yeast. They are considered "super foods," as they can boost levels of protein, vitamins, minerals, energy, chlorophyll, and GLA.[430] Investigate first, then consult with your doctor to see if they'd benefit you during pregnancy or breastfeeding.)

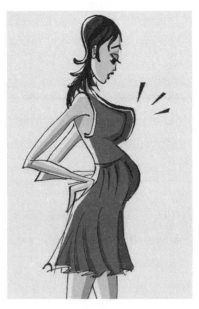

Chapter Fourteen

Breastfeeding:
Suck It Up and Do It

If you only heed one suggestion of ours in this whole entire book, let it be this one: Breastfeed, breastfeed, breastfeed. There is literally nothing you can do that is more beneficial to your baby's immediate and long-term health. And nothing would make us happier than boasting 100 percent of our readers go on to breastfeed their babies.

According to scientific research, studies, and data collection, breastfed babies have higher IQs; better visual acuity;

fewer ear infections; less diarrhea and constipation; less eczema; lower heart rates; fewer instances of pneumonia, influenza, and gastrointestinal and urinary tract infections; and fewer and less severe upper respiratory infections. (Not only does breast milk strengthen immunity in babies, but it also assures a better response to vaccinations.) These lucky tots are also less likely to need tonsillectomies, appendectomies, and even orthodontics! The list goes on. Babies who are breastfed have a decreased risk for childhood cancers (leukemia and lymphomas), juvenile rheumatoid arthritis, diabetes (types I and II), Crohn's disease, ulcerative colitis, food allergies, high cholesterol, obesity,[431] and asthma.[432] Some studies even suggest that breastfeeding can reduce risk of SIDS (sudden infant death syndrome).[433]

Read that list again. And let it sink in. It's not some bullshit, hippie-dippy propaganda. It's science. Whether or not you breastfeed is one of the most important decisions you'll make in your entire life. So don't let a simplistic thought, like, "Well, plenty of babies are formula-fed and they turned out fine," cloud your judgment.

Mother Nature is much craftier than any chemist. While today's formulas have been designed to mimic breast milk as closely as possible, they are no substitute for the real thing. Every time manufacturers add a new component to formulas in an attempt to make them more like breast milk, new components of breast milk are discovered.[434] Pediatric nutrition researchers quoted in *Endocrine Regulations* said it best: "It is increasingly apparent that infant formula can never duplicate human milk. Human milk contains living cells, hormones, active enzymes, immunoglobulins, and compounds with unique structures that cannot be replicated in infant formula."[435]

True that. For starters, the milk a mother produces on day one isn't the same milk she produces on day thirty, or three or six or twelve months in—it's continually changing to meet her baby's needs. It's truly amazing. "First milk" (also known as colostrum, which precedes actual breast milk) is like pure magic for newborns. It's loaded with antibodies to increase immunity and keep fresh, new babies safe from infections. In addition, it creates a protective barrier-like coating on their mucous membranes—in their intestines, noses, and throats.[436] Actual breast milk, which comes in after colostrum, changes during feedings, starting off as thirst-quenching and then becoming hunger-satisfying. Hell, it even adjusts to account for special circumstances: The milk of moms who give birth prematurely contains different amounts of specific nutrients than the milk of moms who carry to term.[437] In comparison to formula-fed preemies, breastfed preemies have fewer blood infections and meningitis,[438] and usually leave the NICU (neonatal intensive care unit) faster.[439]

Breast milk encourages the growth of *helpful* bacteria, which can inhibit the growth of *harmful* bacteria and parasites. One such good bacteria, lactobacillus, is found at levels *ten times* higher in breast-fed babies than in those fed formula. Breast milk is also much easier on babies; they can digest it into their stomachs within fifteen minutes. Formula can take up to sixty minutes![440] Poor babies!

BOOBS EXIST FOR A REASON

We hope that all of you are planning on breastfeeding. But for those of you who aren't, imagine your newborn baby screaming in pain from an ear infection or stomachache. Imagine listening to your baby wheezing and fighting for air. Or God forbid, imagine being told that your child has cancer. We know for some of you, the thought of using your boobs may seem unnatural. But what you need to understand is, the whole reason you've been carting boobs around your entire life is so you could nurse your young! All the other stuff—looking good in clothes, attracting a mate, sexual pleasure—that was just filler to get you to this point. Whether you have small boobs, big boobs, saggy boobs, perky boobs, or lopsided boobs, they are perfectly designed for breastfeeding. (BTW: Size does not matter when it comes to breastfeeding.) Try and let go of whatever feelings you have attached to them and just accept them for the natural wonder they are. And don't be dismissive of breastfeeding simply because you decided way back when you weren't going do it. Just open your mind to it. Don't think we're being bitches and just giving you grief. We truly care about your babies, and we want what's best for them. We also want what's best for you.

BE SELFISH: BREASTFEED!

Of course, what's good for baby is good for mommy. For starters, breastfeeding releases oxytocin into the body. It's a hormone, triggered by the baby's sucking, that causes contractions of the uterus. Yes, this makes your uterus shrink back to normal size faster, but it's also Mother Nature's way of ensuring new moms don't hemorrhage after delivery.

(Moms who opt to bottle-feed are given synthetic oxytocin intravenously, immediately after giving birth. However, hemorrhage risk is still high for 24–48 hours, at which time no oxytocin is administered.)[441] Oxytocin, which is released in your body every time you nurse, also promotes relaxation and nurturing, both of which are vital to moms.[442]

And the last thing any new mom wants is to be laid out for weeks after delivery. Breastfeeding moms are faster to recover from childbirth and less likely to experience postpartum bleeding. It's also been reported that breastfeeding moms are less anxious and more confident than their bottle-feeding counterparts. Maybe one of the reasons is they don't have to worry about birth control! Exclusive breastfeeding can delay the return of your period for 20–30 weeks, which not only reduces the risk of anemia, but also the likelihood of getting pregnant again! When you breastfeed exclusively for six months (and you don't get your period), it's 98 percent effective in preventing pregnancy! And you'll probably be feeling a whole lot sexier—breastfeeding mamas are more likely to return to their pre-pregnancy weights. (You'll also have a reduced risk for long-term obesity.)[443] While this may seem like a matter of vanity, it's actually really important for your health. A woman who gains weight after her first pregnancy is at higher risk for complications like preeclampsia, gestational diabetes, and stillbirth during her second pregnancy.[444] Now granted, you may be having so much heartburn and morning sickness that you never plan on being pregnant again after this. But you certainly want to be around to see your baby become a gown-up. Breastfeeding reduces your chances of developing ovarian and pre-menopausal breast cancers. The longer you breastfeed, the more beneficial.[445] (The same goes for endometrial cancer.)[446]

BREAST IS BEST

Enough about you, you narcissist. Not only do formula-fed babies have longer durations of reflux episodes (spit-up),[447] they're also at an increased risk for tooth decay. (The good bacteria in breast milk fight the bad bacteria that cause tooth decay.)[448] Bottle-fed babies are also at a disadvantage when it comes to speech. According to the *Journal of Pediatrics,* "Early weaning may lead to the interruption of proper oral motor development provoking alterations to the posture and strength of the speech organs and harming the functions of chewing, swallowing, breathing, and articulation of speech sounds. The lack of physiological sucking on the breast may interfere in the oral motor development, possibly causing malocclusion [bad positioning of the upper and lower teeth in relation to each other], oral respiration, and oral motor disorders."[449] Another study in the *Journal of Pediatrics* addresses inguinal hernias, which can affect both sexes, but are ten times more common in males. It is not entirely known why breastfed babies have significantly fewer inguinal hernias. But it could be because breast milk has gonadatropin-releasing hormones, which affects the fetal development of testicles.[450] But boys aren't the only sex to benefit from the breast. Girls who are breastfed (even if only for a short time) have a 25 percent lower risk of developing pre- and postmenopausal breast cancer than girls who are formula-fed.[451]

FORMULA TOTALLY SUCKS

We're sorry, but what lame-ass excuse could you still possibly have for not wanting to breastfeed? Do you think that formula is more convenient? Nothing could be further from the truth. For starters, you need to make sure every bottle, bottle liner, and nipple are sterile each and every time. And in addition to the cost of buying all those supplies, the cost of formula alone can run you about $1,200 per year.[452] You also need to make sure you always have formula on hand, measure the exact amount of water, and heat the bottle to the perfect temperature (all while your baby screams and cries), *and* be 100 percent certain that your water source is free of contaminants. Not to mention the stress of worrying about microwaves (the actual waves themselves, not the ovens) and the agonizing decision over which formula is the healthiest for your baby. As argued in the *Journal of Human Lactation*, "Formula-fed infants depend on products which can be quite different from each other, but which are continually being found deficient in essential nutrients.... These nutrients are then added, usually after damage has occurred in infants or overwhelming market pressure forces the issue."[453] Most compelling of all, no one ever issued a recall on breast milk. But between 1982 and 1994 alone, there have been 22 recalls on infant formula! Seven of those were classified as potentially life threatening! Among the contaminants: pieces of glass, salmonella, and Klebsiella pneumoniae[454] (a bacteria that can cause serious cases of pneumonia)![455] In 2000, Nestlé recalled approximately *three million* cans of formula because, according to the FDA, "The product was manufactured under conditions which suggested that the product may have received a process less than commercially sterile."[456] In 2003, nearly one and a half million cans of formula were recalled under twenty different labels. Reason: "Products may be contaminated with Enterobacter sakazakii,"[457] a rare bacteria that causes high death rates in infants.[458] If that's not enough to keep you up at night, consider the possible implications of using plastic bottles to feed your baby! Multiple independent tests found bisphenol A (BPA), a chemical that mimics estrogen, in plastic baby bottles. According to advocacy group Environmental California, when five of the most popular brands of polycarbonate (clear, shatterproof plastic) bottles were heated, BPA seeped out.[459] With a chemical that mimics estrogen, there is the threat of endocrine disruption, which can cause reproductive problems, interference with hormones, upset to normal development,[460] can affect puberty, and potentially lead to breast and prostate cancers.[461] Genetic damage is also a major concern, which can result in birth defects, mental retardation, and spontaneous abortion for future generations.[462]

All this . . . or . . . you can just lift up your shirt. (Not to mention, you get to eat an additional 300–500 calories a day!)[463]

Breast milk is free, always on tap, and it comes in the perfect temperature. And when your baby needs to be fed in the middle of the night, you don't need to get up, go downstairs, and start measuring, mixing, and heating stuff. You just throw a boob at the kid. It's a no-brainer. Especially for diabetic moms, since breastfeeding often leads to a reduction in insulin and other diabetic medication. Good news all around: Breastfeeding moms tend to have higher HDL levels— "good" cholesterol! This might be the clincher right here: Just the act of producing milk burns up to 500 calories a day! In order to burn off the equivalent, bottle-feeding moms would need to either bicycle for more than an hour or swim thirty laps![464] Part of the weight gained when you're pregnant is an "energy deposit." In other words, you got some chunk on your bod to meet the high caloric demand of nursing.[465] So if you don't breastfeed, you'll actually have to "work" to get rid of the extra chunkage. Need we say more? Fine, we will. Breastfeeding, especially when you switch back and forth from breast to breast, optimizes hand eye coordination.[466] (For the baby, not you.) It also greatly enhances emotional attachment and forges a near-instant bond every time. Bear in mind, you may not feel an immediate connection to your baby the moment he or she is born. As much as moms hate to admit it, it sometimes takes a while for them to really, truly, deeply, and genuinely love their babies. For many, the moment of truth often comes while nursing. It's a truly unique bond that is an honor for you to share. (But just so you know, you can also bond over your strong bones! Breastfeeding decreases chances of osteoporosis for you *and* your baby!)[467]

You can also bond over how eco-chic you are. Every year, in the United States alone, 550 million cans of formula are sold![468] That's just for one year and just in the United States! Imagine all the land, water, energy, and fuel it takes to grow the crops to feed the cows for their milk. Then imagine all the fuel it takes to transport the crops to the cows. Then imagine all the land, water, energy, and fuel it takes to support the cows. Then imagine all the fuel it takes to transport the milk to the pasteurization plants. Then imagine all the energy it takes to pasteurize the milk. Then imagine all the fuel it takes to transport the milk to the factories where they produce the formula. Then imagine all the land, water, energy, and fuel it takes to grow and transport the grains and other additives used in formula. Then imagine all the land, water, energy, and fuel it takes to make the packaging and labeling for the formula.

Then imagine all the fuel it takes to transport all the formula to all the stores. Then imagine all the fuel it takes for all the people to get to the stores to buy the formula. Then imagine all the water it takes to mix with 550 millions cans of formula so that babies can have bottles. Then imagine all the fuel or energy it takes to heat all the bottles. Then imagine all those 550 million empty formula cans sitting in landfills for hundreds of years. Then imagine all the fuel and energy used for the production of plastic bottles, bottle liners, and nipples. Then imagine all the chemicals used in all those processes that are polluting our air, land, and water. Then imagine all the bottles, bottle liners, and nipples sitting in landfills for hundreds of years. Then imagine that you could have curbed all this environmental devastation by breastfeeding your child. Good for baby. Good for you. Good for the environment.

STILL NOT CONVINCED?

Yeah, it's pretty depressing, and we don't blame you for wanting a drink. But the only thing sadder than contributing to the destruction of our planet is opting out of breastfeeding so you can start drinking again. Get it together, sister! Seriously, no judgment here, but if drinking is a motivating factor in deciding whether or not to nurse, you've got a real problem. Run, don't walk, to an AA meeting. To find one near you, visit www.alcoholics-anonymous.org. Yes, there's an old wives' tale about alcohol boosting your milk supply. It happens to be bullshit, so don't even try it! Drinking may make your breasts feel like they're full, but it's just an increase in prolactin, the hormone that stimulates milk supply. But alcohol can actually reduce the amount of milk you produce *and* cause a delay from the time your baby starts sucking until milk is released. And of course, the alcohol you drink gets passed to your baby.[469] If thoughts of smoking are infecting your brain, there are plenty of online resources to help combat those thoughts, too. But so we're clear, nicotine gets passed to your baby through breast milk. When it breaks down into the body, it's known as cotine, and cotine is concentrated in breast milk. In fact, studies showed cotine appearing at levels *three times* higher in breast milk than in mothers' bloodstreams. Not only are you risking allergies, asthma, chest problems, and respiratory disease for your baby, but you're also predisposing him or her to a cigarette addiction like yours.[470] Please, don't let your addictions continue to rule your life and decision-making. You can beat them, but you really need help. Please get it immediately.

And for all you junk-food addicts who just want to go on a Bon Bon bender, it's not gonna get you out of breastfeeding. Yes, it's vital to eat well while nursing—you need to properly nourish yourself and your baby. But if you don't, your baby will still get what he or she needs. The nutrients will just get taken from your body! According to the experts at La Leche League, even in poor countries with cases bordering on malnutrition, mothers who feed on demand have milk that adequately satisfies the needs of their children.[471] That doesn't mean you should eat crap. It just means that if you do have a bad day of eating, you don't need to stress out or feel bad about it.

But make no mistake, caffeine, high fructose corn syrup, coffee (even decaf), soda (diet and regular), refined sugar, and highly processed foods will do you no good. If you drink lots of fresh-squeezed juices and water, you probably won't even want that crap! Not only does fluid help keep your milk flowing, but a lot of moms report feeling thirsty while nursing. So get in the habit of having a glass of water handy every time you nurse.[472]

EATING FOR MILKING

So what should you eat while breastfeeding? Guess! You got

it: A variety of fruits, veggies, nuts, seeds, legumes, and whole grains. Just pay attention to what you eat and when your baby seems fussiest or gassiest. A lot of new moms find journaling really helpful for this. Write down what you eat each day and the times your baby is being an asshole. If you see a pattern, cut the food out of your diet for a full week so it's totally out of your body. Then, with your doctor's blessing, reintroduce it again. If your baby has a brat attack, you'll know which item was to blame. You may not have to give it up forever. Just take a break from offending foods for the first few months of nursing. This will give your baby's gastrointestinal tract more time to develop. Sometimes, unfortunately, really healthy foods can cause gas pains in babies. So keep on the lookout for drama with beans, broccoli, Brussels sprouts, cabbage, cauliflower, citrus fruits, cucumbers, garlic, onions, and peppers. This doesn't mean you should eschew them right from the start—they may be totally fine. Just be conscious of any negative reactions from your baby. (Um, sorry, but there's also a chemical in chocolate that can be a gastric irritant.) And be aware that the most common allergens are dairy products, eggs, wheat, corn, fish, peanuts, nuts, and soy.[473] (Cows' milk and dairy products are at the top of the list, with more than twenty different substances known to trigger allergies in humans.)[474] If you, your husband, or any of your immediate family members suffers from one of these allergies, your child may be susceptible, too. So talk to your doctor before eating these foods. If one of these foods makes your baby seems fussy or gassy, or gives him diarrhea, rashes, hives, the sniffles, or the pukes, let your doctor know and don't eat it again without her "okay."[475]

And check with your doctor to see what, if any, supplements you should be taking. Even though breast milk contains DHA in small amounts, many women now take DHA supplements,[476] which is a good idea. And vegetarians and vegans should take B-12 and D. So be sure your doctor knows your diet and can address your needs accordingly. But something you can probably teach her: vegetarian and vegan women have lower levels of environmental pollutants (like PCBs) in their breast milk than their omnivorous counterparts.[477] Nearly all breast milk is "contaminated" by environmental pollutants, but it is still the healthiest food for babies and should be the number one choice. (Even if you eat meat and dairy.)

HOW LONG IS THIS GONNA TAKE?

For six months, breastfeeding should be the only choice. According to the World Health Organization in collaboration with UNICEF, "Breastfeeding is an unequalled way of providing ideal food for the healthy growth and development of infants; it is also an integral part of the reproductive process with important implications for the health of mothers. As a global public health recommendation, infants should be exclusively breastfed for the first six months of life to achieve optimal growth, development, and health. Thereafter, to meet their evolving nutritional requirements, infants should receive nutritionally adequate and safe complementary foods while breastfeeding continues for up to two years of age or beyond. Exclusive breastfeeding from birth is possible except for a few medical conditions, and unrestricted exclusive breastfeeding results in ample milk production."[478] Now, we can already hear some of you groaning, "Two years? I have to breastfeed for two years?" Pipe down. There's no point now in obsessing about how you're going to feel two years from now. It's like buying a dress today and marking your calendar to wear it two years away. Stay present. And if two years makes you break out in hives, know that the American Academy of Pediatrics recommends, "Exclusive breastfeeding for approximately the first six months and support for breastfeeding for the first year and beyond as long as mutually desired by mother and child."[479] So at the very least, commit to one year. You can do that! If you don't approach it as something that's going be a pain in the ass and you instead embrace it with an open mind, you just might be surprised by how much you love it.

MAKE IT WORK

Yes, plenty of women have horror stories about sore nipples, engorgement, and insufficient milk. But billions more nurse successfully. It's easy to be all keyed up about nursing—we get it. So much is at stake and you really want it to work . . . so much that you're all tensed up, clenched up, and insane about it. Hardly the ideal state to encourage "let down." Just relax. And don't put pressure on your baby or yourself to get it on the first, second, or tenth try. Just breathe. Try different positions. Take breaks if you get frustrated. And don't let your roller coaster emotions take over like a drama queen twelve-year-old. Remember when you learned how to ride a bike? You probably didn't get the concept of balance on the first try. It took a while. And you fell a few times. And more than likely, you didn't "get it" while you were throwing a tantrum. It was only through calm, focused perseverance that you eventually learned. And once you really grasped it, you could hop on and ride anytime, without even thinking about how to balance. It became second nature. It will be just the same with breastfeeding. So expect some scraped elbows and bruised knees, followed by the bliss of riding "no hands." You'll get the hang of it in no time. By the way, unless you're giving birth in a forest all by yourself, you'll have plenty of people to help you learn the ropes. Nowadays, most hospitals and birthing centers have a lactation consultant, whose sole job is to help new moms get comfortable with nursing. Also, the nurses are well versed in the ways of the breast and are all too happy to help. And don't be shy about asking your breast-feeding friends and family for help. Your boobs are gonna be flapping around all the time. Get over it.

Don't have the support of your husband when it comes to breastfeeding? Well, sorry, but he's just a dumb-ass. Perhaps when you tell his dumb-ass that breastfed babies have less offensive diapers, he'll come around. It's true. Breast-milk poop has almost no odor, especially in comparison to formula-poop.[480] That shit is nasty!

What if you want to nurse but the baby has sucking issues?

Well, first, make sure you get help from the lactation experts. If they can't help, try the goddesses at La Leche League (www.LaLecheLeague.org). If they can't help, pump. Breast milk is magic, even if it's in a bottle. Do whatever you can.

So what if you have to go back to work? Nurse at home and pump at the office! Let your boss know that breast-milk babies (even if they're bottle-fed) get sick less often. Translation: If he or she cooperates with your pumping needs, you won't need to miss work for visits to the pediatrician or to take care of a sick baby.[481] Another benefit of pumping is that other family members, like your dumb-ass husband, can share in the joy of feeding the baby. That, and you can go out and have fun and leave the whiny brat with someone else! Yeehaw! (If you know you won't be able to nurse or pump for the long haul, breast-feed for as long as you can—even if it's just for a month, a week, or even a day. Whatever you can do is worth doing. FYI: Experts advise against introducing bottles in the first few weeks. Breastfeeding is the best way to ensure your milk comes in well, continues doing so in adequate amounts, and that your baby gets the hang of the whole thing.)[482]

Yes, there are occasions when a new mom's breasts are engorged and she simply can't "let down" her milk. But typically, if you're having trouble breastfeeding, it's not a medical problem. It's usually related to improper positioning, stress, exhaustion, anxiety, insecurity, embarrassment, resentment, fear of pain, or negative comments from ignorant family members or friends.[483] So if you're really struggling, know that there's likely nothing wrong with you, and that you just need some quiet, peaceful, patient, alone-time with your newborn. But if you desperately want to breastfeed, have tried everything, and are still unable, do not beat yourself up. You are NOT a failure, you are still a good mother, and your baby will be fine. Make peace with the situation and don't allow yourself to get depressed.

PLAN B

There are alternatives. What if you have a medical situation that prevents you from producing milk but you want your baby to have the benefits of breast milk? What if you can't nurse and your baby has medical problems that will be exacerbated by formula? Now, try and stay with us, because it's gonna sound totally off the wall and maybe even kinda gross to some of you: milk banks. Altruistic women, who are carefully screened and tested, donate their breast milk. And both the American Academy of Pediatrics and La Leche League endorse the safety of milk banks.[484] Do a google search for "milk banks." Many doctors don't even know donated milk is an option, yet there are milk banks all over the world. It's okay if the nearest bank is miles away; they can overnight frozen milk to you. Most legitimate places require a doctor's prescription and many charge fees (approximately $3.50 per ounce + shipping—it depends on the place) to offset their costs. It can be expensive, considering infants can consume 20–30 ounces a day. However, some insurance plans will cover these costs. Regardless, be sure you're only soliciting legitimate, safe, ethical milk banks. Buying milk from the cheapest place, some random online broker, or a stranger you met on craigslist is not the way to go, and it can be unsafe. (Conversely, paying top dollar doesn't ensure safety, either.) Check out the standards of the Human Milk Banking Association of North America at www.hmbana.org. In addition to their many guidelines, they only accept milk by donation, meaning, they don't pay women for their breast milk. Those who donate to them are motivated solely by the urge to help others. Offering money for milk could invoke unscrupulous behavior in those with skewed intentions.

We know it sounds entirely crazy to accept the breast milk of a human stranger, but is it really crazier than getting udder milk from a cow stranger? Really. Take a moment to think about why one sounds weird and the other normal. And then see if you can reverse the two. Yes, the idea will take getting used to, especially since our society equates breasts with sex more than breastfeeding. But isn't every child's health more important than tiptoeing around societal taboos? Whether you think you'll need it or not, it wouldn't hurt to do some quick research on milk banks and discuss donated milk with your husband. It would behoove you both to know what your options are and have an agreement on what you'll do should the need arise. And if the need does arise, be sure to work with your doctor in finding a safe and trusted source.

PLAN C

Hopefully, your foray into the world of milk banks will just be thought provoking and theoretical, because you'll breastfeed with ease and enjoyment. And hopefully you won't want or need to supplement with formula. There is so much conflicting information on which is "better"—soy or cow's milk—that it had us reeling. And we knew you'd be looking to us to sort it out for you. Well, we're sorry to say, the whole thing is just one big mess.

According to Susan Baker, MD, former chair of the AAP Committee on Nutrition, "Parents can feel confident that soy-based infant formulas are safe. For over fifty years, millions of babies have grown and developed normally on soy-based formulas. Mother's milk is the best nutrition for babies. The American Academy of Pediatrics policy is that soy formulas are safe and effective for babies who are not being breast-fed and cannot tolerate a cow-milk formula."[485]

So in their eyes, soy formula is an acceptable alternative if your baby cannot tolerate cows' milk formula. But if you paid attention during the dairy chapter, you'll remember all the diseases cows' milk and dairy products are associated with: heart disease; diabetes; obesity; osteoporosis; kidney stones; cataracts; macular degeneration; multiple sclerosis; Alzheimer's; and breast, prostate, colon, and rectal cancer![486] Do we think we're smarter than the entire medical community that comprises the American Academy of Pediatrics? No. But would Kim give her son cows' milk formula knowing what she knows about cows' milk? Hell no. Does Rory plan on giving her future children cows' milk formula? No way. (She's well aware she needs to get a boyfriend first.)

Having said that, are either of us stoked about soy formula? Not entirely. But in its defense, it's *not* associated with all the evils of dairy. All the concerns about soy are speculative. And allergies to soy protein are less common than allergies to cows' milk protein.[487] (God, it must have killed the National Dairy Council to admit to that!) Also, immune responses to the proteins in cows' milk have been implicated in type-I diabetes and Sudden Infant Death Syndrome (SIDS)![488] Opponents of soy formula express concern that phytoestrogens could increase risk of endocrine-sensitive cancers and could have adverse effects on fertility and sexual development.[489]

However, these concerns are based on animal studies, which scientists agree cannot be accurately correlated to human studies. Additionally, a long-term study comparing infants who drank soy formula and milk formula found no significant differences between the two groups in more than thirty outcomes related to growth, development, reproduction, and other health issues. It was reported that, statistically, soy-fed females menstruated for approximately eight hours longer with somewhat more discomfort. However, according to the study's authors, "The results with regard to menstruation should be interpreted with caution, given that the clinical significance of slightly prolonged menstrual bleeding in the absence of greater menstrual flow is not known. Given the large number of comparisons evaluated in these analyses, the few marginally significant findings may be due to chance. Although perhaps these few marginal positive findings should be followed up in future studies, the findings of the current study are reassuring about the safety of soy infant formula."[490] We'd be more reassured if the study wasn't financed in part by the International Formula Council. But the U.S. Department of Agriculture's chief scientific research agency is funding another long-term study (six years) on the matter.[491] However, it won't be complete until September 2008, a year after we hand this manuscript in to our publisher. (Don't be writing to us in October 2008 to ask what the outcome is! Start taking matters into your own hands and research it yourself. Go to www.ars.usda.gov and do a search under "Arkansas Children's Nutrition Center" and "soy-based infant formula." And if that doesn't work, try some variation. Figure it out.)

We are both huge believers in breastfeeding and would do whatever it took to make it work. And if we couldn't give our children our own breast milk, we would likely aim for human milk from another source. Now, we know you'll want to know what we would do if we were in a pinch and *had* to pick between soy formula and cows' milk formula. And we hesitate to tell you because we're not doctors, research scientists, or anything of the sort. (We also want you to think for yourselves.) But we know if we don't tell you, you'll flood us with annoying e-mails, so here goes. If we needed the odd bottle of formula on occasion, we would choose soy. But again, that is just for an occasional supplement to breastfeeding under extenuating circumstances. And it's just the personal choice of two broads who have no formal education in obstetrics, pediatrics, or epidemiology. So to reiterate, we would both breastfeed, first and foremost. If we couldn't, we would likely aim to obtain human breast milk from another source. And on the rare occasion when we were in a pinch and needed to supplement, we would choose soy over cow formula. (Please note: Soymilk and soy formula are entirely different from one another and soymilk should **never** be used in place of soy formula.)

But for heaven's sake, would you just breastfeed your child, please.

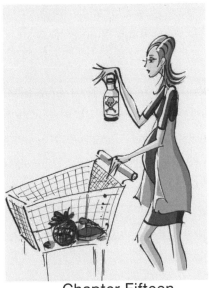

Chapter Fifteen

The Companies You Trust Don't Care About Your Children

The party's over, ladies. You're responsible for another life now, so the days of blissful ignorance have come to an end. You cannot trust others to keep you safe. From this moment on, you need to read the ingredients of every single thing you buy. And we're not just talking about food, because manufacturers of baby products and beauty products will screw you, too!

There are about 1,700 new chemicals entering the market-place every year, and they're almost entirely untested.[492] Laboratory tests released in February 2007 revealed the presence of one carcinogenic chemical, 1,4-Dioxane, in multiple children's bath products. And we aren't talking some obscure products you've never heard of. We're talking bath products sold by Hello Kitty, Huggies, Sesame Street, Gerber, Disney, Scooby Doo, Rite Aid, Lil' Bratz, L'Oréal Kids, and Johnson.[493] This will surely come as a shock to you (it shocked us): The FDA has no legal authority to require companies to assess the safety of their cosmetics. And, according to Jeanne Rizzo, RN, executive director of the Breast Cancer Fund (a founding member of the Campaign for Safe Cosmetics), "Because the FDA does not require cosmetic products to be approved as safe before they are sold, companies can put unlimited amounts of toxic chemicals in cosmetics."[493] That includes baby products! The FDA works with manufacturers on a *voluntary* basis.[494] Wow! How reassuring! Companies can voluntarily adhere to the FDA's recommendations ... or not.

The United States has outlawed eight ingredients for cosmetic use. The European Union has banned more than one thousand! Phthalates, a family of chemicals, are among the forbidden in the EU, but they are legal in the United States.[495] Commonly found in beauty products, food packaging, vinyl, plastics, baby books, teethers, bath toys, and other toys, phthalates have been linked to asthma[496] and developmental and reproductive health risks.[497] A small study published in *Environmental Health Perspectives* found that pregnant women with the highest levels of phthalates in their urine had sons with subtly altered genitals (including slightly smaller penises and testicles that didn't descend completely).[498] We'd tell you to avoid them at all costs, but companies aren't always required to disclose their presence! And sometimes, even when companies claim their products are phthalate-free, they aren't.[499]

Our skin is our largest organ. And because it has all those countless pores, everything we put *on* our skin gets *under* our skin. So unless you'd want it coursing through your bloodstream and getting processed by your organ systems, don't put it on your skin. The skin of babies is even more permeable than our own, and their brains, nervous systems, and organs are still in development. So they're especially vulnerable to chemicals in products.[500] Which is why it's pretty disappointing when brand names you've known and trusted for decades turn out to be completely unconcerned with consumer health. Actually, it's pretty disgusting. How any company can put profits before people (especially babies) is beyond us. But it's rampant, nonetheless. Just to name a few, as of September 2007, Pampers Baby Fresh Diaper Wipes contain Dimethicone, iodopropynl butylcarbamate, sodium hydroxymethylglyanate, BIS-PEG, and fragrance; Gerber's Grins & Giggles Lavender Baby Wash has disodium lauroamphodiacetate, cocamidopropyl betaine, PEG-80, PEG 150 distearate, Quarterium-15, D&C Violet #2, and D & C Red #33; and Johnson's Baby Lotion has methylparaben, propylparaben, butylparaben, BHT, fragrance, and Red #33![501] Huggies has the audacity to market baby wipes in a "Natural Care" line and list their ingredients as "gentle ingredients." These "natural" and "gentle" ingredients include potassium laureth phosphate, polysorbate 20, tertrasodium EDTA, DMDM Hydantoin, and methylparaben. What the hell are these things and all the other crap found in baby/beauty/skincare products? Oh nothing much. Just a bonding agent that could not only irritate skin, but possibly even burn it; a formaldehyde-releasing preservative; carcinogens; allergens; endocrine disruptors; and chemicals that can cause an increased risk of breast cancer, reduced fertility, pregnancy complications, neurotoxicity, immunotoxicity, organ system toxicity, developmental/reproductive toxicity, and irritation to the eyes and lungs.[502] Imagine having a bottle of poison with a skull and crossbones on it. Then, someone adds a cream base to it, along with some color and a pretty smell. They slap a label over the skull and crossbones, you buy it, and slather it all over yourself to avoid stretch marks (or on your baby to heal diaper rash). Nicely done. Those days are over. Read the ingredients, read the ingredients, read the ingredients. Of everything. And if you don't know what something is, find out. (That doesn't mean e-mailing and asking us.)

Stay away from acne medications, especially Accutane, and anything that contains retinoic acid, retinol, or any other retinoid—they can cause birth defects. As can some anti-aging/wrinkle/night creams, which often contain large amounts of animal-derived vitamin A.[503] Things that contain benzoyl peroxide and salicylic acid are also considered unsafe during pregnancy,[504] and some experts caution against alpha-hydroxy acids (AHAs).[505] When you're breastfeeding, pay special attention to your boobs. Only wash them with water (no soap). And if you're having nipple issues, don't just automatically reach for the nipple cream. For starters, your baby will be eating it! But regardless, do you really want to add a product filled with chemicals to a vulnerable area of your body? Why are we so programmed to medicate and treat everything with chemicals, like it's the most normal thing in the world? We need to retrain our brains here. Using your own breast milk as a moisturizer is the best thing you can do. Really. But if that doesn't cut it, try a little organic coconut or olive oil from your kitchen, some natural, fragrance-free shea butter, or a combination of the three. However, be aware that even though commercial nipple creams can contain these ingredients, there's always the possibility of infant allergens. So check with your healthcare provider first, and then, regardless of what you apply, make sure you wash it off thoroughly before nursing. We'd offer you some suggestions for good nipple creams, but were hard-pressed to find ones without vitamin E and lanolin. Some experts say not to use vitamin E, because it isn't safe for babies to ingest and it often comes in a wheat germ oil base (wheat is a potential allergen.)[506] And lanolin is the grease off a sheep! (Eew! Gag, gag, gag!) Imagine finding a hairy, smelly, greasy guy, and then taking his dreadlocks and squeezing them between rollers to get the grease out. Then imagine rubbing that grease on your boobs! (Or on your lips, because lanolin is in a lot of lip balms!) Puke, gross, nasty! A lot of "natural" books and websites will suggest lanolin, but in addition to it being revolting, there's also the risk of pesticide and antibiotic residue. Not good for your boobs and not good for your baby. So stop being hung up on the idea that you need some bottled, fragrant, colored lube to heal sore, dry, or cracked nipples. Start thinking outside the box and use natural home remedies, like olive oil, coconut oil, or shea butter. And if you insist on buying a bona fide nipple cream, just go to a store (or a website) that sells natural products, pick out a few that catch your eye, and read the ingredients. (Even if we did recommend a brand or two, you still need to get in the habit of reading ingredients. Manufacturers sometimes change their formulas. So a product that received high marks at some point may now be on our shit list.)

Even disposable diapers are a toxic nightmare; they're filled with shit before you even put 'em on your baby! According to the Environmental Protection Agency, dioxin (a highly toxic by-product of bleaching) and other dyes can cause damage to the kidneys, liver, and central nervous system. Sodium polyacrylate, the absorbent gel in diapers, has been linked to toxic shock syndrome, allergic reactions,[507] skin irritations, and respiratory problems.[508] Considering it can also be very harmful and even potentially lethal to pets,[509] are we supposed to feel good about putting it against our babies' genitals twenty-four hours a day, just so we can keep them dry? We recommend using organic cloth diapers or buying organic disposables. (FYI: Children who wear cloth diapers often potty-train earlier than those in disposables. Without all the crazy chemicals, cloth diapers aren't as absorbent, so children can feel the discomfort of when they're wet and learn faster.[510])

And as New Age as it sounds, we also recommend getting your baby an organic mattress. Phthalates are common in conventional baby mattresses. And because polyurethane foam, the predominant filling material, is essentially solid petroleum, mattresses are very flammable. So manufacturers add toxic flame retardants. The most common, pentaBDE, is associated with hyperactivity and other neuro-behavioral problems. It doesn't adhere to the foam, so it leaches out into the surrounding air, occupied by your sleeping newborn. Polyvinyl chloride (PVC), one of the most toxic and reviled of all, is the surface material used in almost all baby mattresses.

It too is treated with flame retardants. In addition to all that jazz, your baby is likely getting chemical catalysts, surfactants, emulsifiers, pigments, formaldehyde, benzene, toluene, and other chemical additives, as well.[511] Because your baby spends between ten and fourteen hours a day sleeping, and every breath she takes will be no more than six inches away from this chemical shit-storm, we recommend investigating natural, organic baby mattresses and bedding. (It wouldn't hurt to get yourself some good sleeping gear, too.) P.S. Infant sleep accessories made of foam (like sleep wedges and positioners) can also be treated with toxic flame retardants. And again, even those labeled "phthalate-free" are often not.[512] So really research and crosscheck everything you buy. Don't just take the manufacturer's word for it.

If you're engaged enough to put a bow in her hair or match his sneakers to his onesie, you can take the time to make sure you're not poisoning your child. So when you start adding food to your baby's regimen, we expect nothing but diligence from you! Gerber, Beech Nut, and Heinz account for more than 95 percent of all baby food sold in the United States, with Gerber having 70 percent all to itself.[513] So you'd think the industry front-runners must be doing something right to corner the market the way they do. You'd think. But the truth is, parents suck at reading labels. Because if they were better informed, they'd be choosing other brands! All four of Heinz's toddler cereals—Nutrios, Apple Cinnamon Crisps, Blueberry Crisp, and Mixed Berry Crisps—have sugar in them![514] Sugar! There's no reason on the planet for a toddler to have sugar. None. Let's say you feed him something you make yourself, and there's no sugar in it. And he clearly likes it and eats the whole thing. Then let's say you feed him something with sugar in it. Now you've given him a taste for it, and eventually, the sugar-free version won't be as palatable. So you'll be thinking, "Gee, Jimmy just loves Heinz's cereals so much." Yeah, 'cause there's friggin' sugar in it. It's one thing when your kid gets older and he's surrounded by sugar everywhere. But when he's a baby or toddler and you can easily control everything he eats, there's no reason for sugar to be on the menu! Or salt, for that matter! The American Academy of Pediatrics recommends that salt not be added to baby foods,[515] yet a call to Gerber's 800 number revealed that their third stage Broccoli & Carrots with Cheese and their second stage Macaroni & Cheese Dinner both have salt.[516] Their Graduates line also had some doozies: The Meat Sticks

are made of pork, beef, salt, and sugar. (Um, is there anything
in there actually good for a child?) The Diced Green Beans
have salt, the Sweet Corn Puffs have sugar, the Zwieback
Toast has sugar and partially hydrogenated cottonseed oil,
the Juice Treats have corn syrup as the first ingredient, and
the Cereal Bars have sugar, high fructose corn syrup, and
modified corn starch! Ask yourself why manufacturers would
put those kinds of ingredients in any food, let alone baby
food. Did you ask yourself? What answer came to mind? If
they aren't motivated by money, we don't know what they're
motivated by. Because there is no acceptable justification for
putting sugar, high fructose corn syrup, or hydrogenated oil
in baby food. Baby food should be packed with fresh, organic,
wholesome ingredients and nothing else. But Beech Nut
seems to think watering down their foods is the way to go.
In their stage two Four Delicious Dinner Varieties (Macaroni
& Beef with Vegetables, Sweet Potatoes & Chicken, Turkey
Rice Dinner, and Chicken & Rice Dinner), water is listed as
the second ingredient in every single dish. So you get to pay
for less food, and your baby gets to eat less nutrients. Great,
huh? Ladies, we give you the three top-selling baby food companies in the United States: Gerber, Heinz, and Beech Nut.

Making your own baby food is not rocket science. It's just as easy as cooking and mashing. Done. Remember, *Skinny Bitch: Bun in the Oven* is a book for how pregnant women should eat plus a few extras here and there. So don't be complaining that we don't give you four weekly menus for your kid's food. Read books and study up on how and what to feed your baby. *Vegetarian Pregnancy and Baby Book* by Amanda Grant is a good resource. (Just ignore any dairy references. Gross.) And if you insist on being too lazy to make your own, buy organic baby food. But still read the ingredients!

You and your baby are going to be eating as purely as possible. And all your "beauty" products will be as natural as possible. So it'd be counterproductive to go fumigating your house with all sorts of toxic, industrial cleaners. Vinegar, water, and baking soda can clean almost anything. And there are plenty of natural cleaning products on the market, too. But don't just buy something that says "natural" on the bottle. Read the ingredients and educate yourself.

The Complete Organic Pregnancy by Deirdre Dolan and Alexandra Zissu is a good resource for learning about home and beauty products. And the Environmental Working Group has a great database for cosmetic and personal care products: www.cosmeticsdatabase.com. But feel free to poke around and look for your own resources. Because from now on, you've got to be a savvy consumer. Your baby's counting on you.

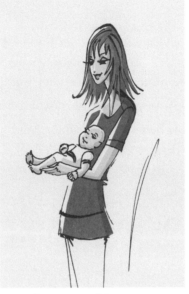

Chapter Sixteen

Post Push

Congratulations! You're a mommy! And now that you've gone through labor, you can handle anything. Even a little post-delivery bleeding, which is totally normal. Lochia (pronounced lo-kee-ah) is when blood, tissue, and mucus are expelled from the uterus. (Gross, sorry.) It can last for two weeks or two months, and will be bright red, then pink, then brown, then yellow, and then clear.[517] (Oh, so gross. Sorry.) Don't be alarmed. Just slap in a pad and go about your business. (No tampons allowed.) But if you soak a pad in less than an hour, are bleeding bright red after seven days, have a fever or chills, or have a funky-smelling discharge, go to the doctor ASAP.[518]

All right, on to greener pastures. Like how crazy you're gonna be. While you may consider your offspring as the second coming of Christ, let us put things in perspective for you: You are his or her mother, not his or her God. It is your job to feed, clothe, comfort, care for, and protect your baby. It is not your job to be perfect or saintly or divine. You are human. And this will be the hardest job you'll ever have in your entire life. Of course, it will also be the most rewarding, but there will be many times when you are sleep-deprived, cranky, exhausted, overwhelmed, hormonal, impatient, irritable, and otherwise imperfect. Accept it. Embrace it. Be prepared for it. We can already hear some of you clucking to yourselves, "Not me. I'm gonna love my baby. When he's fussing, I'll be soothing and patient and nurturing. I'll know just what to do. I was born to be a mom." Get your head out of your uterus and wake up! Motherhood is going to kick your ass. And there's nothing wrong with that, because you're human, remember? So long as you're not disillusioned about it, you'll be fine. So when you're having a bad day, or even a few strung together, remember what we said: It is your job to feed, clothe, comfort, care for, and protect your baby. So in those moments when your freshly diapered, recently fed, just-bathed baby is crying for no $%#@ reason for the third night in a $%#@ row when all you want is one night of $%#@ sleep . . . and for that split-second you don't love your baby—forgive yourself. You're not a bad mom. You're human. And your baby is a total monster.

Being human translates to other areas of your life, too, even if you're Superwoman now. Get over the need to be perfect. Managing life around the demands of a feisty newborn isn't easy. It'll take time to adjust, so again, let go of the notion that you'll be different than all the other moms who struggle.

No mom is an island. So let others help you. If too much time with your own mom makes your skin crawl, be specific: "Mom, would you come over tomorrow from 12 pm to 3 pm? You can see the baby and help me get some stuff done, if you wouldn't mind." And when she comes, don't hog the baby. It's easy to have that God-complex, like you're the only one who can do "it" right. Whether it's feeding, burping, changing, holding, or calming the baby—there is more than one way to do things. So allow others the privilege of loving your baby.

You may learn something. Just the act of letting go will be really beneficial for you. It'll make you realize that you can still have a life *and* a baby.

This will be a great test to see how you really regard your husband. Many women think their husbands are completely clueless and incompetent when it comes to babies. And many men are. But that's because the women in their lives never allow them to learn the ropes. It takes time to get comfortable doing anything new. Handling a baby is no different. So don't act like the baby is yours or huff and tsk when he tries to bond with his newborn. Let him be a dad. Be moved by it. He's the only other person on the planet who'll love the child as much as you do. And he's the only other person on the planet who'll listen to your boring monologues about how special and beautiful and precious your baby Jesus is.

Because none of your friends will want to hear it. Your friends *without* kids will want to shoot themselves every time you open your mouth. So it's vital you make mommy friends. They won't care when you go on and on about junior. They'll just tune you out—until it's their turn to talk about their little miracles. New moms are like clucking hens. And they're cooped up alone all day with their newborns, just dying to talk to someone. It's easy to feel isolated, lonely, and even depressed, sometimes. Making friends that are able to relate to your circumstances can make the entire experience more enjoyable. Seriously. Do you want your baby spending her formative years in a shroud of silence? Or do you want her surrounded by people and energy and life? Don't think that it's your little family vs. the whole world. You'll lose. And your marriage will suffer. Having friends makes a woman more interesting and lively and fun. Bonus: Mommy friends are the best resources for pediatricians, schools, and about ten million helpful hints.

They're also good to exercise with. When your healthcare provider gives you the go-ahead, get active. It's not healthy for anyone to live a sedentary life. So don't let being a mom serve as an excuse to avoid exercising. Obviously, you put on weight when you're pregnant. If you don't take charge, that extra weight will become a permanent fixture. You don't need to start training for a marathon, just get off your ass and go outside. Walking and talking and pushing your stroller will likely be the highlight of your day. Fresh air, sunlight—good for you, good for baby. You'll get your heart pumping, your milk flowing, and your uterus shrinking. You'll start to feel like a person again, and not just a host body. You'll also get those endorphins going, which can combat any "baby blues" you might feel. All this will help you feel good about yourself, regardless of how much you weigh.

Exercise is great for all that and more. But now is not the time to become fanatical about losing weight or getting in shape. You just had a baby! And it was a tremendous burden physically. Don't tax your body further with some crazy-ass exercise regimen. You'll do more harm than good. Exercise with your baby because it feels good and allows you to spend time with that little love-monkey. But don't be an image-obsessed lunatic. Who wants a mom like that? Remember, it took you nine months to gain all that weight. So give yourself a reasonable amount of time to lose it.

Regardless, don't let the weight get you down. It'll be hard enough if you have to battle the "baby blues" or postpartum depression; the last thing you need is to feel bad about your body. About 70 to 80 percent of women experience the baby blues—mood swings, irritability, fear, anger, and unexplained crying spells. You're tired all the time, you feel slightly over-whelmed, and you aren't entirely in love with your kid just yet.[519] All normal. And temporary. Thankfully, after about two weeks or so, the baby blues are usually gone. But an unlucky 10 to 20 percent of moms actually have postpartum depression (PPD). The difference between the two? PPD can last significantly longer and/or feel significantly worse. It's basically clinical depression that occurs sometime after giving birth.[520] PPD is characterized by:

- Feeling like a failure.
- Feeling disinterested in, detached from, or negative about your baby.
- Feeling so tired you can't get out of bed for days and can't take care of your baby.
- Thinking about hurting yourself or your baby.[521]
- Excessive worrying about your baby's health.
- Obsessive thoughts about your baby's safety.
- Trouble falling asleep, waking up extremely early, or sleeping too much.
- Having an abnormally small or large appetite.
- Having little to no energy.
- Having reduced sex drive and dysfunction. (Cut yourself some slack here. A baby just came out of your lady pocket.)
- Feeling hopeless, like you'll never feel better.[522]

Now, don't start panicking that your head is going to spin around like in *The Exorcist*, but a very small percentage of women can also experience postpartum psychosis, accompanied by anxiety attacks, paranoia, delusions, hallucinations, confusion, suicidal thoughts, and a lost grasp on reality. But acute cases like these are more likely to strike those with a history of bipolar disorder, so fear not.[523]

Whether you have the baby blues, PPD, or you're stark raving mad, it's not your fault! After birth, there are dramatic drops in your estrogen and progesterone levels; your thyroid level can also drop; and there can be differences in your blood pressure, immune system functioning, and metabolism.[524] No wonder you go a little batshit! Who wouldn't? But if you feel like you have PPD or worse, don't think you're Superwoman and you can do it all alone; get help right away. Call your doctor ASAP. Women suffering from PPD are less likely to recognize and react to their babies' cues. This can cause "insecure attachment," which may have negative and long-lasting effects on your baby. Children of depressed moms are at higher risks for behavioral, social, and emotional problems; delays in cognitive development; and depression.[525]

While it's good to be prepared for anything, don't resign

yourself to having the baby blues or PPD. There are a few things you can do to reduce the chances of having either. For all you working moms: One study found that those who took 12 weeks of maternity leave (as opposed to 6 weeks) had 15 percent fewer PPD symptoms after going back to the office.[526] So see what you can work out. Maybe if you tell your boss you'll be less likely to go postal at the office ... Also, studies have suggested that breastfeeding can decrease the likelihood of PPD and/or lessen its impact. Additionally, weaning slowly, as opposed to abruptly, can reduce your risk.[527] Exercising, adhering to your old routine as much as possible, and carving out some alone time are also good tools in your arsenal. After you nurse your baby, hand him or her off to your husband, lock yourself in the bathroom, and take a nice, quiet bath.[528] (Or lock yourself in the bedroom and take a nap!) Whatever you need, allow yourself the luxury. Small things can go a long way in making you feel like a civilized member of society again.

But probably the most useful trick of all: clucking like the hen you are! Women are social creatures. We need each other. We need to tell each other our problems and know we aren't alone. Simply being heard and understood can make all the difference in the world. So reach out to your friends, family members, and even that lummox of a husband. It wouldn't hurt to warn him about PPD ahead of time, so he knows what to look for, how serious it is, and doesn't say anything stupid like, "Can't you just snap out of it?" Let him know you'll need him to really help out with baby care, house chores, and anything else that might overwhelm you in your delicate state. And instruct him on how to best serve you as a friend during that time. "Honey, I'm gonna vent to you, and I don't want you to try and 'fix it' or make it better. I just want you to empathize, offer your support, and be extra loving." And keep that friggin' wiener of yours the hell away from me!

It's totally normal to lose interest in sex for a period of time after delivering. Most new moms have sex 75 percent less often than they did prior to getting pregs. So tell your husband it's only temporary and to back it the hell up. (Then give him a bottle of hand lotion and run!) At some point, though, you're gonna have to sleep with your husband again. Typically, doctors recommend waiting six to eight weeks after delivery. So if you need more time, make up a different number. But know that most first-time parents do it two to three times a month after the eight-week mark.[529] Pervs.

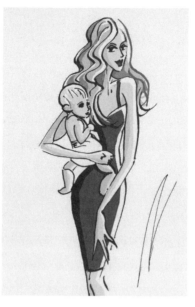

Chapter Seventeen
What Makes a M.I.L.F.?

There's a term that young, single guys use for sexy moms: M.I.L.F. It's an acronym for Mother I'd Like to #$%@. Don't be insulted; it's the highest compliment a stupid man can pay you. (And don't be frightened. It's always muttered behind your back. No man would ever be so bold as to tell you to your face.) You can pretend to be shocked, appalled, and offended, but you're not fooling anyone. There will come a time when you're feeling unattractive and loathsome—you'll be wearing your fat pants for the tenth consecutive week, you'll be covered in spit-up, and you'll have likely gone weeks without so much as a nod from your husband. One day, when you take the pains to doll yourself up and you catch an appreciative glance from a hot young buck, you'll remember: "I've still got it." It'll put a spring in your step. And it'll raise the bar for you to get it together on a more regular basis.

Not just in the looks department, though. (A woman who overvalues her appearance is a bimbo—mother or not.) You'll be inspired to be a whole person again, and not just a mommy. Remember what it was like before you became a mom? When you had ideas, thoughts, and opinions about things other than your child? Having outside interests or personal needs doesn't make you a bad mom. It makes you human. Nurturing those needs and interests will make you a better mom. If you're feeling resentful or unfulfilled or bored, you're of no use to your baby. In fact, you suck for your baby. She never asked you to become a single-minded, lame-ass bore. So quit blaming her. She'd prefer to have a happy mom with a rich, layered life. She can survive without you for an hour a day, or for as many hours as you need to feel happy and whole. Don't use motherhood as an excuse to give up on your own life. It's an easy trap to fall into. So be strong.

And be vigilant. Don't be a sucker for advertising anymore. Read the labels of everything you buy. If you're going to put it in your mouth or on your skin, or in your baby's mouth or on her skin, you better know exactly what it is. No ifs, ands, or buts. Use your own head and don't believe or trust anyone. Do your own research and make your own well-informed decisions. You're a big girl now.

And love yourself, big ass and all. Mommies who love themselves make babies who love themselves. Good health is the most important thing you can give your baby. Confidence is the most important thing you can instill in your child. And you can't instill it in your kid while you're busy knocking yourself. Would you ever allow your daughter to think her self-worth is tied up in her body? Would you adore and worship her any less if she were chubby? So why do you deserve less than your daughter? Be the type of woman you want her to be. Or raise the kind of man you'd want a daughter to marry. Do you want your son to choose a supermodel or a super girl? One of them is fool's gold.

Now just because looks are unimportant, that doesn't mean you shouldn't honor and celebrate yourself. Buy cute clothes for your sexy mommy body and rock your new curves. Get over the, "I still need to lose X pounds" bullshit and just have fun. Don't put being happy and confident on hold until your scale reads a specific number. Be happy and confident now! It's not an external thing. It's simply a choice. And if you'd open your eyes, you'd recognize that there are few things more beautiful than confidence. Confidence is at the pinnacle of beauty, along with generosity, gratitude, and love.

You're a mother now. It is an honor and a gift to give life. Feel nothing but blessed by the miracle that has been bestowed upon you. Bask in the glow. And extend your love to not only your child, but to all children. And in fact, embrace all moms, who are really no different than you. While you're at it, love those who are childless. Hell, you might as well love everyone. What greater purpose can you serve than to love everyone? What greater lesson can you teach your child than to love everyone? What greater way can you better the world than to love everyone in it?

Mahatma Gandhi said, "Be the change you wish to see in the world." If you can embody that, you won't ever have to teach your child anything. You can just be.

Works Cited

"AAP Releases Revised Breastfeeding Recommendations." Aap.org, Feb. 7, 2005; accessed Sept. 9, 2007, http://www.aap.org/advocacy/releases/feb05breastfeeding.htm

"A Cesspool of Pollutants. Now Is the Time to Clean-Up Your Body." Nealhendrickson.com. August, 2004; accessed on Mar. 6, 2007, http://www.nealhendrickson.com/mcdougall/ 2004nl/040800pucesspool.htm

"Alert: Another Sneak Attack on Organic Standards: USDA to Allow More Conventional Ingredients in Organics." Organicconsumers.org; accessed Sept. 9, 2007, http://www.organicconsumers.org/articles/article_5225.cfm

"Alert Update." Organicconsumers.org; accessed Apr. 6, 2007, http://www.organicconsumers.org/epa6.cfm

Andersson, Ingrid. "Food-Borne Risks in Pregnancy." Willystreet.coop. April 2005; accessed Nov. 21, 2006, http://www.willystreet.coop/newsletter/Newsletter_Archive/0504/ midwife.html

"Animal protein & fat raise endometrial cancer." Reuters.com. *International Journal of Cancer*. Apr. 15, 2007; accessed Sept. 10, 2007, http://www.reuters.com/article/healthNews/iduscol16846020070321

Apuzzo, Matt. Associated Press. "Judge allows private testing for mad cow disease in U.S." Organicconsumers.org, Mar. 30, 2007; accessed Sept. 9, 2007, http://www.organicconsumers.org/articles/article_4655.cfm

Arcoverde, Denise. "World Breastfeeding Week. Breastfeeding: Nature's Way." Waba.org, 1997; accessed Sept. 9, 2007, http://www.waba.org.my/wbw/wbw97/afonline.htm

Artal, Raul, Rosemary B. Catanzaro, Jeffrey A. Gavard, Dorothea J. Mostello, and Joann C. Friganza. "A lifestyle intervention of weight-gain restriction: diet and exercise in obese women with gestational diabetes mellitus." *Applied Physiology, Nutrition, and Metabolism*. 32(3): 596–601 (2007) doi:10.1139/H07-024. Date modified Sept. 12, 2007, accessed Sept. 12, 2007; http://pubs.nrc-cnrc.gc.ca/cgi-bin/rp/rp2_tocse?apnm_apnm3-07_32

"Ask the Fitness & Nutrition Experts." Babyfit.com, updated Sept. 5, 2007; accessed Sept. 14, 2007, http://babyfit.sparkpeople.com/ask-the-experts-answers.asp?inID=80%20

"Aspartame: What You Don't Know Can Hurt You." Mercola.com; accessed Jan. 21, 2007, http://www.mercola.com/article/aspartame/hidden_dangers.htm

"Aspartame: What You Don't Know Can Hurt You. Natural Ingredients Imply 'Not Harmful" Mercola.com; accessed Jan. 21, 2007, http://www.mercola.com/article/aspartame/not_natural.htm

"Baby Alert: Why Plastic Teethers & Bottles Are Bad." Ecowise.com. April 21, 1999; accessed May 21, 2007, http://www.ecowise.com/information.php?info_id=21

"Baby blues or postpartum depression." Mommysmunchkins.com; accessed Sept. 13, 2007, http://www.mommysmunchkins.com/depression.php

"Baby Care Products." From *The Learning and Developmental Disabilities Initiative*. Jan. 2007. Iceh.org; accessed Sept. 10, 2007, http://www.iceh.org/pdfs/LDDI/PracPrevention/BabyCareProducts.pdf

"Back pain during pregnancy." Mayoclinic.com. Jan. 20, 2005; accessed Nov. 15, 2006, http://www.mayoclinic.com/print/pregnancy/HQ00302/METHOD=print

"Bacteria Enterobacter Sakazakii." Reference.com, last updated Mon. Jun. 11, 2007; accessed Sept. 9, 2007, http://www.reference.com/browse/wiki/Bacteria_Enterobacter_Sakazakii

Barnard, Neal, MD. *Breaking The Food Seduction: The Hidden Reasons Behind Food Cravings—and 7 Steps to End Them Naturally.* New York: St. Martin's, 2003.

Barnard, Neal, MD. "Meat Too Tough to Eat." Pcrm.org, published in *Hartford Courant*, accessed Sept. 14, 2007, http://www.pcrm.org/news/082806.html

Barnes, Lisa. *The Petit Appetit Cookbook: Easy, Organic Recipes to Nurture Your Baby and Toddler.* New York: The Penguin Group, 2005.

Barnes, Liza. "Maternity Leave Helps Banish the Baby Blues." Babyfit.com. Updated Sept. 5, 2007; accessed Sept 10, 2007, http://babyfit.sparkpeople.com/articles.asp?id=753

"Beauty Dos & Don'ts for Pregnant Women." ivillage.com; accessed Dec 5, 2007, http://beauty.ivillage.com/0,,j1ph,00.html

Beck, Leslie, R.D. *The Ultimate Nutrition Guide for Women.* Original edition by Pearson Education Canada: 2001.

"Benefits of Breastfeeding." Drgreene.com; accessed May 9, 2007, http://www.drgreene.com/21_552.html

"Benefits of Breastfeeding." Usbreastfeeding.org; accessed May, 2007, http://www.usbreastfeeing.org/Issue_Papers/Benefits.pdf

Bernstein, Henry, M.D. "Soy Formula as Alternative to Breast Milk." Life.familyeducation.com; accessed Sept. 10, 2007, http://life.familyeducation.com/baby/nutrition/40669.html

Bierma, Paige. "Getting to the Bottom of Pregnancy Cravings." Caremark.com, accessed May 10, 2007, http://healthresources.caremark.com/topic/printview

"Birth Defects." Clevelandclinic.org.; accessed Sept. 13, 2007, http://www.clevelandclinic.org/health/healthinfo/docs/3800/3811.asp?index=12230

"Birth Defects and Pharmaceutical Drugs." Oshmanlaw.com; accessed Sept. 12, 2007, http://www.oshmanlaw.com/personal_injury/birthdefects.html

"Birth Defect Statistics." Pcrm.org; accessed Nov. 21, 2006, http://www.pcrm.org/resch/charities/statistics.html

Blaauw, R. et al. "Risk factors for development of osteoporosis in a South African population." *SAMJ*–1994; 84:328–332.

"Breast Milk Interactions Charts." Babycenter.com; accessed May 18, 2007, http://www.babycenter.com/general/8788.html

Booth, Hobson, MD, ACOG, and Mary Lynn Alpino. "Exercise During Pregnancy Helps You Stay Healthy." Firstbabymall.com; accessed May 18, 2007, http://www.firstbabymall.com/expecting/pregnancy/exercise.htm

Bouchez, Colette, Reviewed by Louise Chang, MD. "Pregnancy Skin Care: Get That Glow." Webmd; accessed Dec. 5, 2007, www.webmd.com/baby/features/pregnancy-skin-care-get-that-glow

"Bovine Spongiform Encephalopathy." Wikipedia.org, last modified Sept. 7, 2007; accessed Sept. 9, 2007, http://en.wikipedia.org/wiki/Mad_cow_disease

Boyles, Salynn. "Weight Gain Between Pregnancies Increases Risks." Foxnews.com. Friday, Sept. 29, 2006; accessed May 18, 2007, www.foxnews.com/printer_friendly_story/0,3566,216661,00.html

"Breastfeeding Benefits from Top to Bottom." Askdrsears.com; accessed May 9, 2007, http://askdrsears.com/html/2/T020300.asp

Brown, Harold. E-mail to Rory Freedman, Mar. 21, 2005.

Burby, Leslie. "101 Reasons to Breastfeed Your Child." Promom.org. May 2005; accessed May 19 2007, http://www.promom.org/101

Burch, Elizabeth, N.D., and Judith Sachs. *Natural Healing for the Pregnant Woman*. New York: A Lynn Sonberg Book. A Perigee Book. Published by The Berkley Publishing Group, 1997.

"Bush EPA Nominee Abandons Insecticide-on-Children Study After Senate Hearing." Wikinews.org, Apr. 9, 2005, last modified Jun. 3, 2007; accessed Sept. 9, 2007, http://en.wikinews.org/Bush_EPA_nominee_abandons_insecticide-on-children_study_after_Senate_hearing

"C-Section: Medical Reasons." Marchofdimes.com, April 2006; accessed Sept. 9, 2007, http://www.marchofdimes.com/pnhec/240_1031.asp

"Caffeine." Counseling Sheets. Ucheepines.org; accessed Sept. 12, 2007, http://www.ucheepines.org/caffeine.htm

"Caffeine Facts." Shapefit.com; accessed Sept. 12, 2007, http://www.shapefit.com/caffeine-effects.html

Campbell, T. Colin, PhD, and Thomas M. Campbell II. *The China Study: Startling Implications for Diet, Weight Loss and Long-Term Health*. Dallas, TX: Benbella Books, 2006.

"Cancer-Causing Chemical Found in Children's Bath Products." Campaign for Safe Cosmetics. Feb. 8, 2007; accessed Sept. 10, 2007, Environmental Working Group, http://www.ewg.org/files/14-dioxane.pdf

"Causes of Shortness of Breath During Pregnancy." Marchofdimes.com; accessed Nov.15, 2006, http://www.marchofdimes.com/pnhec/159_16046.asp

Challem, Jack. "Caution Urged with Vitamin A in Pregnancy—But Beta-Carotene is Safe." From the *Nutrition Reporter Newsletter*, 1995; accessed Sept. 9, 2007, http://www.thenutritionreporter.com/A-vitamins.html

Chandel, Amar. "Sweet Poison," *The Tribune Spectrum*, March 14, 2004; accessed March 22, 2005, www.tribuneindia.com/2004/20040314/spectrum/main1.html

Chavarro, Jorge E., M.D., Walter C. Willett, M.D., and Patrick Skerrett. "Fat, Carbs, and the Science of Fertility." *Newsweek*, December 10, 2007, 58.

"Chlorpyrifos." Wikipedia.org, last modified Aug. 25, 2007; accessed Sept. 9, 2007, http://en.wikipedia.org/wiki/Chlorpyrifos

Cik, Barry A. PE, CP, DEE, QEP, REM, CHMM. "Five Problems with Baby
    Mattresses (toxic chemicals)." Healthychild.com; accessed Sept. 12, 2007,
    http://www.healthychild.com/toxic-chemicals-baby-mattress.htm

Clark, Nancy, MS, RD. "The Athlete's Kitchen. Roughing-up Your Sports
    Diet." Princeton.edu. May 2003; accessed Mar. 21, 2007,
    http://facilities.princeton.edu/Dining/_Nutrition/The_ATHLETE_Kitchen
    05_03.htm

"Constipation." Healthynj.org; accessed Mar. 21, 2007,
    http://www.healthynj.org/dis-con/constipation/main.htm

"Constipation during pregnancy." Health-cares.net, accessed Mar. 21, 2007,
    http://digestive-disorders.health-cares.net/constipation-pregnancy.php

"Constipation During Pregnancy." Solutions.psu.edu, 2006; accessed Mar. 21,
    2007, http://solutions.psu.edu/Nutrition_Fitness_575.htm

"Consumers Union and OCA criticize USDA for Latest Appointments of
    So-Called "Consumer Representatives" to the National Organic Standards
    Board." Organicconsumers.org, Jan. 19, 2005; accessed Sept. 9, 2007,
    http://www.organicconsumers.org/SOS/critics011906.cfm

Cook, Christopher D. "Environmental Hogwash: The EPA Works with Factory
    Farms to Delay Regulation of Extremely Hazardous Substances" Oct. 6,
    2004; accessed Jan. 27, 2005,
    www.inthesetimes.com/site/main/print/environmental_hogwash

Core, Jim. "Study Examines Long-Term Health Effects of Soy Infant Formula."
    Agricultural Research Magazine, Jan. 2004; accessed Sept. 10, 2007,
    http://www.ars.usda.gov/is/AR/archive/jan04/soy0104.htm

"Cosmetics and Anti-Aging Products—What's Safe During Pregnancy?"
    Womenshealthcaretopics.com, accessed Dec. 5, 2007,
    www.womenshealthcaretopics.com/bn_bodysoul_cosmetics_pregnancy.htm

Coupe, Kevin. "Editorial: Mad Cows, Lunatic Politicians, & the Case for
    Traceback." Cattlenetwork.com, May 1, 2006; accessed Sept. 9, 2007,
    http://www.cattlenetwork.com/content.asp?contentid=33332

Cousens, Gabriel, M.D. *Conscious Eating*. Berkeley, CA: North Atlantic Books, 2000.

"Cow's Milk Allergy versus Lactose Intolerance." *National Dairy Council*. Vol. 77, No. 3 May/June 2006; accessed Sept. 10, 2007, http://www.national-dairycouncil.org/NationalDairyCouncil/Health/Digest/ded77-3Page1.htm

"The Cost of Preeclampsia in the USA." Preeclampsia.org; accessed Sept. 9, 2007, http://preeclampsia.org/statistics.asp

Cropper, Carol Marie. "Does It Pay to Buy Organic?" Businessweek.com. Sept. 6, 2004; accessed Mar. 13, 2007, http://www.businessweek.com/magazine/content/04_36/b3898129_mz070.htm

Cumming, R. G., Klineberg, R. J. "Breastfeeding and other reproductive factors and the risk of hip fractures in elderly woman." *Int J Epidemiol* 1993; 22:684–691

Cummins, Ronnie. "Congress Allocates $5 Million for Organic Farming Research." Organic Trade Association, May 23, 20006; accessed Sept. 9, 2007, http://www.organicconsumers.org/2006/article_534.cfm

Curtis, Glade B, MD, OB/GYN and Judith Schuler, MS. *Your Pregnancy Week by Week*. 4th Ed. Cambridge, MA: Da Capo, 2000.

"Dairy Products Linked to Parkinson's Disease." PCRM online e-mail subscription. Pcrm.org; accessed Jun. 25, 2007

Davis, Brenda, RD and Vesanto Melina, MS, RD *Becoming Vegan: The Complete Guide to Adopting a Healthy Plant-Based Diet*. Summertown, Tenn: Book Publishing Company, 2000

Davis, Karen, PhD. *Prisoned Chickens Poisoned Eggs. An Inside Look at the Modern Poultry Industry*. Summertown, TN: Book Publishing Company, 1996.

DeFao, Janine. "Glass baby bottles making comeback. Stores selling out after health alarms raised about plastics." Sfgate.com. Monday, April 9, 2007;

accessed May 27, 2007, http://www.sfgate.com/cgibin/article.cgi?file=
/c/a/2007/04/09/BOTTLES.TMP

DeFao, Janine. "Moms pay big for other mothers' milk. But doctors warn non-
nursing women of health risk to babies." *San Francisco Chronicle*. Sun Apr.
9, 2006; accessed Sept. 8, 2007, http://sfgate.com/cgibin/article.cgi?f=
/c/a/2006/04/09/ MNGLKI6FTA1.DTL

Delany, Richard M, MD, FACC, "Omega-3 Fat During Pregnancy."
DrDelany.com, accessed March 6, 2006,
http://www.drdelany.com/Preventive_Updates_2004_test_51.asp?patient=

DeNoon, Daniel J. "Danger in Plastic Baby Bottles?" Webmd.com. March 31,
2003; accessed May 27, 2007,
http://www.webmd.com/baby/news/20030331/danger-in-plastic-baby-bottles

Dermer, Alicia, MD., IBCLC, and Anne Montgomery, M.D. "Breastfeeding:
Good for Babies, Mothers, and the Planet." Medicalreporter.health.org;
accessed May 9, 2007,
http://medicalreporter.health.org/tmr0297/breastfeed0297.html

Desjardins, Ellen, MHSc, RD. "Just Say No to a Low Carbohydrate Diet."
Todaysparent.com, Autumn 2000; accessed Nov, 2006,
http://www.todaysparent.com/pregnancybirth/nutrition/article.jsp?
content=4046&page=1

De Wals, Philippe PhD., Fassiatou Tairou, MSc, Margot I. Van Allen, MD, Soo-
Hong Uh, MSc, R. Brian Lowry, MD, Barbara Sibbald, MSc, Jane A. Evans,
PhD, Michiel C. Van den Hof, MD, Pamerla Zimmer, MHSA, Marian
Crowley, MN, Bridget Fernandez, MD, Nora S. Lee, MSc, and Theophile
Niyonsenga, PhD. "Reduction in Neural-Tube Defects after Folic Acid
Fortification in Canada." *The New England Journal of Medicine*. Jul. 12,
2007: 135

"Diapers, Diapers & More Diapers. Cloth vs. Disposable." The newparents-
guide.com; accessed Sept. 10, 2007, http://www.thenewparentsguide.com/
diapers.htm

"Does It Pay to Buy Organic?" For pregnant women and children, the benefits are worth the higher price." Business Week, Sept. 6, 2004; accessed Sept. 14, 2007,http://www.businessweek.com/magazine/content/04_36/b3898129_mz070.htm

Dolan, Deirdre, and Alexandra Zissu. *The Complete Organic Pregnancy: What You Need to Know—From the Nail Polish You Wear to the Bed You Sleep in to the Water You Drink*. New York: Collins, 2006.

Donohoe, Martin, MD. "Letter to the Editor of Wall Street Journal: Long-standing Evidence of rBGH Dangers." Organicconsumers.org. Feb. 7, 2007; accessed Feb. 9, 2007, http://www.organicconsumers.org/articles/article_4034.cfm

Donovan, Debbi, IBCLC. "Postpartum depression: Can nursing lessen its impact?" ivillage.com; accessed Sept.9, 2007, http://parentingivillage.com/newborn/ndepression/0,,3x1b,00.html

Douglas, Ann. "Pregnancy Food Cravings: Fact or Fiction." Pregnancyandbaby.com; accessed Mar 2007, http://pregnancyandbaby.com/pregnancy/baby/Pregnancy-food-cravings-fact-or-fiction-61.htm

"Drug-Resistant Bacteria Found in U.S. Meat." *Reuters Medical News*, May 24, 2001

Dunley, Ruth. "Smoking ruins breast milk. The equivalent of 20 cigarettes can be passed on to infants." Apparenting.com; accessed May 19, 2007, http://apparenting.com/smoking-while-nursing.html

Durocher, Heather Johnson. "The Low-Carb Craze. Should Pregnant Women Participate?" Pregnancytoday.com; accessed Jan. 31, 2007, http://pregnancytoday.com/articles/2038.php

"E. Coli Infection." Familydoctor.org. American Academy of Family Physicians, updated Sept 2006; accessed Sept. 9, 2007, http://familydoctor.org/242.xml

"Eating Disorders during Pregnancy." Americanpregnancy.org; accessed Sept. 9, 2007, http://www.americanpregnancy.org/pregnancyhealth/eatingdisorders.html

"Eating for Two: Weight Influences on Pregnancy." Americanpregnancy.org; accessed Nov 15, 2006, http://www.americanpregnancy.org/pregnancyhealth/eatingfortwo.html

"Eggs Non Gratis." From Autumn 1998 issue of *The Civil Abolitionist*. Web.linkny.com; accessed Mar. 13, 2007, http://web.linkny.com/~civitas/page74.html

Eisenberg, Arlene, Sandee E Hathaway BSN and Heidi E. Murkoff. *What to Expect When You're Expecting*. New York: Workman Publishing, 1991.

Eisnitz, Gail A. "Ask the Experts." Peta.org; accessed Sept. 9, 2007, http://www.goveg.com/vegkit/meet.asp

Eisnitz, Gail. *Slaughterhouse: The Shocking Story of Greed, Neglect, and Inhumane Treatment Inside the U.S. Meat Industry*. Amhers, MA: Prometheus Books, 1997.

"Eleven States Oppose EPA Mercury Proposal." Oag.state.ny.us. Jun. 28, 2004; accessed Apr. 6, 2006, http://www.oag.state.ny.us/press/2004/jun/jun28b_04.html

Elliot, Rose MBE. "Mother and Baby Guide." Viva.org.uk; accessed Nov. 21, 2006, http://www.viva.org/uk/guides/motherandbaby.htm

Environmental Working Group's Skin Deep Cosmetic Safety Database. Cosmeticdatabase.com; accessed Dec. 5, 2007, http://www.cosmeticdatabase.com

"EPA's Latest Human Pesticide Testing Rule Called Illegal, Immoral." Ens-newswire.com; accessed Apr. 6, 2006, http://www.ens-newswire.com/ens/jan2006/2006-01-25-05.asp

Epstein, Samuel, S., MD. *The Politics of Cancer* (Revisited), East Ridge Press, NY, 1998

Epstein, Samuel, MD. *"What's In Your Milk?"* Preventcancer.com; accessed
    Feb. 9, 2007, http://www.preventcancer.com/publications/WhatsInYour
    MilkRelease.htm

"Excessive weight gain during pregnancy directly associated with having an
    overweight child." News-medical.net. Mon, Apr. 2, 2007; accessed May 11,
    2007, http://www.news-medical.net/?id=22856

"Exercising While You're Pregnant." Babyfit.com; accessed May 18, 2007,
    http://babyfit.sparkpeople.com/pregnancy-fitness-guide.asp
"Fantastic Fiber." Askdrsears.com; accessed May 21, 2007,
    http://www.askdrsears.com/html/4/T041500.asp

FDA's Mission Statement. U.S. Food and Drug Administration. Fda.gov;
    accessed Sept. 10, 2007, http://www.fda.gov/opacom/morechoices/
    mission.html

"FDA Recalls of Baby Formula." Breastfeeding.com, accessed Sept. 9, 2007,
    http://www.breastfeeding.com/advocacy/advocacy_recalls.html

Ferdowsian, Hope, M.D, and Susan Levin, R.D. "Fish Still Not a Healthy
    Choice." Pcrm.org. Published in The Providence Journal, Oct. 24, 2006;
    accessed Nov. 21, 2006, http://www.pcrm.org/news/commentary061024.html

"Fetal Death and Growth Retardation." Georgiastrait.org; accessed Mar. 6,
    2007, http://www.georgiastraight.org/?9=node/643

Fialka, John. "EPA Scientists Pressured to Allow Continued Use of Dangerous
    Pesticides." Organicconsumers.org. *Wall Street Journal* Page A4, May 25, 2006;
    accessed Jun, 2006, http://www.organicconsumers.org/2006/article_540.cfm

Fink, Randy A, MD., FACOG. "Pregnancy weight gain: What to expect."
    Babycenter.com. Last updated Dec 2006; accessed May 11, 2007,
    http://www.babycenter.com/0_pregnancy-weight-gain-what-to-expect_1466.bc

"Fishy Advice." VegNews. March/April 2008, 29

"Food Additives/Preservatives and Pregnancy." Pregnancyweekly.com; accessed Sept. 14, 2007, http://www.parentingweekly.com/pregnancy/pregnancy_health_fitness/food_additives.htm

"Food cravings and what they mean." Babycenter.com, last reviewed March 2003; accessed Sept. 13, 2007, http://www.babycenter.com/refcap/pregnancy/pregnancynutrition/1313971.html

"Foods Rich in Fiber." ivillage.com. Jan. 1, 2000; accessed Mar. 21, 2007, http://health.ivillage.com/eating/enutritional/0,,m8r-p,00.html

"Free-Range Eggs and Meat: Conning Consumers?" Peta.org; accessed Mar. 16, 2005, http://peta.org/mc/factsheet_display.asp?ID=96

Freni-Titulaer, L.W, J.F. Cordero, L. Haddock, G. Lebron, R. Martinez, and J.L. Mills, "Premature Thelarche in Puerto Rico. A Search for Environmental Factors," *American Journal of Diseases of Children*. 40 (1986): 1263–1267

Freudenheim, J., et al. "Exposure to breast milk in infancy and the risk of breast cancer." *Epidemiology* 1994; 5:324-331

"Full Profile. Nitrite, Nitrate." Checnet.org; accessed Nov. 21, 2006, http://www.checnet.org/HealtheHouse/chemicals/chemicals-detail2.asp?Main_ID=278

Gangemi, Jeffrey. "Start ups Across America. How many new businesses are created each year? A new Kauffman Foundation study tracks entrepreneurial activity in the U.S." Businessweek.com, May 23, 2007; accessed Sept. 9, 2007, http://www.businessweek.com/smallbiz/content/may2007/sb20070523_138444.htm?campaign_id=rss_smlbz

Gates, Donna. "The Surprising Reason You May Be Aging Prematurely: Improper Protein Digestion." Bodyecology.com; accessed Mar. 13, 2007, http://www.bodyecology.com/06/12/21/getting_enough_protein.php

Geller, Robert J, MD, FAAP. "Questions About Pesticides on Foods." *Journal of Medical Toxicology* Volume 2, Number 3. ACMT.NET. Sept. 2006; accessed Dec. 10, 2006

Gelles, Jeff. "Why antibiotics in meat should give you pause." *The Philadelphia Inquirer*. Dec. 11, 2002.

Gerber. Telephone interview. 1-800-4-GERBER. Sept. 12, 2007

"Gestational Diabetes: Causes, Symptoms and Management." Womenfitness.net; accessed Jan. 23, 2007, http://www.womenfitness.net/gestational_diabetes.htm

Gillette, Becky. "Premature Puberty: Is Early Sexual Development the Price of Pollution?" *E: The Environmental Magazine*. Nov. 1997

"Global Strategy for Infant and Young Child Feeding." World Health Organization in collaboration with UNICEF

Gold, Mark. "Common Toxic and Unhealthy Substances to Avoid." Holisticmed.com; accessed Feb. 28, 2005, http://www.holisticmed.com/aspartame/history.faq

Gold, Mark. "Formaldehyde Poisoning from Aspartame." Dec. 9, 1998; accessed Mar. 6, 2005, http://www.holisticmed.com/aspartame/embalm.html

Golding, Jean, PhD, DSc. Email to Rory Freedman, May 3, 2007

Grace, Matthew. *A Way Out: Dis-Ease Deception and the Truth About Health*. U.S.A: Matthew Grace, 2000

Green, Che. "Not Milk: The USDA, Monsanto, and the U.S Dairy Industry." *Lip Magazine*, July 9, 2002; accessed Feb. 20, 2005, http://www.alternet.org/story/13557/

Greene, Alan M.D. "Benefits of Breastfeeding." Drgreene.com, July 21, 1996, last reviewed 2001; accessed Sept. 13, 2007, http://www.drgreene.com/21_552.html

Greenfield, Marjorie, M.D. "Vaginal Infections During Pregnancy." Drspock.com; accessed Nov. 15, 2006, http://www.drspock.com/article/0,1510,5984,00.html

Greenfield, Marjorie, M.D., Lisa Rodriguez, R.N. "Sciatica During Pregnancy." Drspock.com. Aug.21, 2004; accessed Nov. 15, 2006, http://www.drspock.com/article/0,1510,4411,00.html

Greger, Michael, MD. "Paratuberculosis and Crohn's Disease: Got Milk?" Veganoutreach.org; Jan. 2001; accessed Nov. 30, 2006, http://www.veganoutreach.org/health/gotmilk.html

Greger, Michael, MD. "Plant-Based Diets Beneficial in Pregnancy." Drgreger.org; accessed Nov. 30, 2006, http://www.all-creatures.org/health/plantbased-mg.html

Greger, Michael MD. "Mercury Contamination in Fish." Vegetarianbaby.com; accessed Sept. 12, 2007, http://www.vegetarianbaby.com/articles/mercuryfish.shtml

Greger, Michael, M.D. "Vegan Children: A Recent Review." Drgreger.org. Sept, 2004; accessed Nov. 1, 2006, http://www.drgreger.org/september2004.html

Hand, Becky RD. "Figuring Out Fiber Part 1." Babyfit.com; accessed Mar. 21, 2007, http://babyfit.sparkpeople.com/articles.asp?id=505

"Hazardous Chemicals Found in a Wide Range of Baby Products." *Environmental News Service*. Oct. 13, 2005; accessed Sept. 10, 2007, http://www.organicconsumers.org/school/babyprods101405.cfm

Heacock, HJ. "Influence of Breast vs. Formula Milk in Physiologic Gastroesophageal Reflux in Healthy Newborn Infants" Jour. Pediatr Gastroenterol Nutr, 1992 January; 14(1): 41–6 993

"Health news—alcohol lowers breast milk production." Bupa.co.uk. April 18, 2005; accessed May 18, 2007, http://www.bupa.co.uk/health_information/html/health_news/180405 breastfeeding.html

"Here's essential exercise information for pregnant women, plus some gentle postpartum moves." *Fit Pregnancy*. August/September 2006: 124

"Here's to Pickles and Ice Cream." Medicinenet.com. Reviewed Jan. 30, 2005; accessed May 9, 2007, http://www.medicinenet.com/script/main/art.asp? articlekey=51635

Herrick, Kirsten, David I. W. Phillips, Soraya Haselden, Alistair W. Shiell, Mary Campbell-Brown, and Keith M. Godfrey. "Maternal Consumption of a High-Meat, Low-Carbohydrate Diet in Late Pregnancy: Relation to Adult Cortisol Concentrations in the Offspring." *The Journal of Clinical Endocrinology & Metabolism*. Vol. 88, No. 8. Jcem.org, copyright 2003 by The Endocrine Society; accessed Jan. 31, 2007, http://jcem.endojournals.org/cgi/content/full/88/8/3554

Holford, Patrick. *The Optimum Nutrition Bible*. Berkeley: The Crossing Press, 1999

Hooper, Lee, Rachel L. Thompson, Roger A. Harrison, Carolyn D. Summerbell, Andy R Ness, Helen J. Moore, Helen V. Worthington, Paul N. Durrington, Julian P. T. Higgins, Nigel E. Capps, Rudolph A. Riemersma, Shah B. J. Ebrahim, and George Davey Smith. "Risks and benefits of omega 3 fats for mortality, cardiovascular disease and cancer: systemic review." Bmj.com. (*British Medical Journal*). BMJ 2006; 332: 752–760 (Apr. 1); doi: 10. 1136/bmj. 38755.366331.2f. Published Mar. 24, 2006; accessed Sept. 11, 2007, http://www.bmj.com/cgi/content/full/332/7544/752?ehom

Hoops, Stephanie. "Jury still out on plastic baby bottles' safety." Montereyherald.com. May 21, 2007; accessed June 10, 2007, http://www.montereyherald.com/business/ci_5946714

"Hormone 'Replacement' Increases Cancer Risk." *Good Medicine Magazine*, Winter 1998 Volume VII, Number 1. Pcrm.org; accessed Nov. 21, 2006, http://www.pcrm.org/magazine/GM98Winter/GM98Win7.html

"How Breast Milk Is Produced." Sutterhealth.org; accessed May 18, 2007, http://www.babies.sutterhealth.org/breastfeeding/bf_production.html

"How Can I Get Enough Protein? The Protein Myth." Pcrm.org; accessed Mar. 13, 2007, http://www.pcrm.org/health/veginfo/ protein.html

Howell, Edward M.D. *Enzyme Nutrition: The Food Enzyme Concept*. U.S.A.:
    Avery, 1985

Huggins, Kathleen, R.N. "How breastfeeding benefits you and your baby."
    Babycenter.com. June 2005; accessed May 9, 2007,
    http://www.babycenter.com/refcap/baby/babybreastfeed/8910.bc

"IFC Discusses a Study on Soy Infant Formula and Adult Health Outcomes."
    International Formula Council. Infantformula.org. Mar.14, 2006; accessed
    Sept. 9, 2007, http://www.infantformula.org/newsroom_20060314_2.html
"Investigation Reveals Slaughter Horrors at Agriprocessors." Peta.org;
    accessed Mar. 17, 2005, http://www.goveg.com/feat/agriprocessors/

"Is It Safe for My Baby?—Laxatives." Camh.net, accessed Sept. 7, 2007,
    http://www.camh.net/About_Addiction_Mental_Health/Drug_and_Addicti
    on_Information/Safe-Baby/safe_baby_substance_laxative.html8

"Johnson's Baby Lotion." Johnson & Johnson Consumer Companies, Inc.
    accessed Sept 9, 2007, http://www.johnsonsbaby.com/product.do?id=24

Johnson, Kate. "High Sugar, Fat Intake During Early Pregnancy Increases
    Preeclampsia Risk." Findarticles.com. May 15, 2000; accessed Jan. 24, 2007,
    http://findarticles.com/p/articles/mi_m0CYD/is_10_35/ai_62827604

Johnson, Lucy. "Aspartame ... A Killer!" *The Sunday Express*. London, U.K.
    Newfrontier.com; accessed Mar. 21, 2005,
    http://www.newfrontier.com/asheville/aspartame.htm

Jolliffe, Tanya. Ask the Fitness & Nutrition Experts. Babyfit.com. Updated
    Sept. 5, 2007; accessed Sept 8, 2007

Kalwart, H.J., and Specker, B.L. "Bone mineral loss during lactation and recov-
    ery after weaning." Obstet. Gynecol. 1995; 86:26–32

"Kids Safe Chemical Act Empowers EPA to Require Chemical Testing."
    Environmental News Service. Mon. Jul. 18, 2005; accessed Sept 10, 2007,
    http://www.truthout.org/cgi-bin/artman/exec/view.cgi/34/12714

Kirkpatrick, David D. "EPA Cancels Pesticide Tests on Floridian Babies."
    Apparenting.org. Apr. 8; accessed Apr. 6, 2006,
    http://www.apparenting.com/epa_cancels_pesticide_tests_on_floridian_
    babies.html

Klaper, Michael M.D. Pregnancy, *Children and the Vegan Diet*. Hawaii:
    Gentleworld, 1987

Klein, Diane and Rosalyn T. Badalamenti. *Eating Right for Two. Delicious
    Recipes and Menus for Every Day of Every Month*. New York: Ballantine, 1983

Kradjian, Robert M, MD. "The Milk Letter: A Message to My Patients."
    Vegsource.com; accessed Dec. 6, 2006,
    http://www.vegsource.com/articles/kradjian_milk.htm

Landrigan, Philip J. "The Unique Vulnerability of Infants and Children to
    Pesticides." Mindfully.org. EHP v. 107, Supp.3 Hun 99; accessed Mar. 6, 2007,
    http://www.mindfully.org/Pesticide/Children-Infants-Vulnerability.htm

Langeland, Terje. "Tainted Meat, Tainted Money: Consumer groups decry cozi-
    ness between government, agribusiness." *Colorado Springs Independent
    online edition*, Aug. 1-7, 2002; accessed Sept. 9, 2007,
    http://www.csindy.com/csindy/2002-08-01/cover2.html

Lauersen, Niels, M.D., PhD and Colette Bouchez. *Getting Pregnant: What You
    Need to Know Right Now*. New York: Fireside, 1991

Levis, Sophia. "Dealing with Constipation During Pregnancy."
    Amazingpregnancy.com; accessed Mar. 21, 2007,
    http://www.amazingpregnancy.com/pregnancy-articles/29.html

Linden, Ann, CNM. "Vaginal discharge during pregnancy."
    Babycenter.com. Jun 2006; accessed Nov.15, 2006,
    http://www.babycenter.com/refcap/pregnancy/prenatalhealth/270.html

"Link Eyed Between Beef and Cancer. Tests Show Likely Link Between Growth Hormone and Breast Cancer." Cbsnews.com, May 20, 2003; accessed Sept. 9, 2007, http://www.cbsnews.com/stories/2003/05/20/eveningnews/main554857.shtml

"Livestock a major threat to the environment." Fao.org, Nov. 29, 2006; accessed Sept. 9, 2007, http://www.fao.org/newsroom/en/news/2006/1000448/index.html

Loesche, W.J., "Nutrition and dental decay in infants." Am J Clin Nutr 41; 423–435, 1985

"Low-Fat Dairy Products Linked to Increased Infertility Risk." pcrm.org, Mar. 6, 2007; accessed Sept. 15, 2007, http://www.pcrm.org/news/archive070306.html

"Lowey Calls for Hearing on NY's Mercury Pollution as EPA Proposes Rules That Are Too Lax." House.gov. Feb. 10, 2004; accessed Apr. 6, 2007, http://www.house.gov/list/press/ny18_lowey/100204mercuryepa.html

Mangels, Reed, PhD, FADA. "Vegetarian Diets During Pregnancy." Andrews.edu; accessed Feb. 10, 2007, http://www.andrews.edu/NUFS/Vegetarian%20Diets%20During%20Pregnancy.html

Manzella, Debra R.N. "A Fiber-Rich Diet Decreases Risk for Gestational Diabetes." About.com; accessed Mar. 21, 2007, http://diabetes.about.com/b/a/000057.htm

Marino, Sal. "Ten Best Selling Books of all Time." Industry Week. Answers.google.com, July 1999; accessed Sept. 14, 2007, http://answers.google.com/answers/threadview?id=329063

Marshall, Helen. "Over-the-counter medicines in pregnancy." Netdoctor.co.uk. Last updated Apr. 11, 2007; accessed Sept. 13, 2007, http://www.netdoctor.co.uk/health_advice/facts/medicinesinpregnancy.htm

Martin, Andrew. "How to Add Oomph to 'Organic'." Nytimes.org, published
    Aug. 19, 2007; accessed Sept. 9, 2007,
    http://www.nytimes.com/2007/08/19/business/yourmoney/19feed.html?
    ex=1189310400&en=2b9b40776ea0c111&ei=5070

Martini, Dr. Betty. "Report for Schools, OB-GYN and Pediatricians on
    Children and Aspartame/MSG." Wnho.net. Posted Aug. 4, 2006;
    accessed Jan. 21, 2007,
    http://www.wnho.net/report_on_aspartame_and_children.htm

Matthiessen, Connie. "Mommy, Mama, Mutter: Motherhood Around the
    World." Lifestyle.msn.com; accessed Sept. 13, 2007,
    http://lifestyle.msn.com/familyandparenting/raisingkids/articlebc.aspx?
    cp-documentid=4843327&page=1
Maugh, Thomas H. II. "Diet soda, metabolic syndrome linked." LAtimes.com, Jul.
    24, 2007; accessed Sept. 9, 2007, http://www.latimes.com/features/ health/
    nutrition/la-sci-soda24jul24,1,500458.story?coll=la-health-nutrition-news

McNeil, Donald G, Jr. "U.S. Reduces Testing for Mad Cow Disease, Citing Few
    Infections." Jul. 21, 2006; accessed Sept 11. 2007, http://www.nytimes.com/
    2006/07/21/washington/21cow.html?ex=1175918400&en=8

"Meat-Eating Moms Have Less Fertile Sons." Pcrm.org. Posted Apr. 3, 2007;
    accessed Sept. 10, 2007, http://www.pcrm.org/news/archive070403.html

"Meat: Not Suitable for Children." Goveg.com; accessed Mar. 6, 2007,
    http://www.goveg.com/lettuce_meat.asp

Meldung, Nachste. "High protein/low carbohydrate diet when pregnant leads
    to higher stress susceptibility in children." Innovations-report.de. Mar. 4,
    2006; accessed Jan. 30, 2007, http://www.innovations-report.de/
    html/berichte/medizin_gesundheit/bericht-57400.html

Melton, L.J., Bryant, S.C., Wahner, H.W., et al. "Influence of breastfeeding and
    other reproductive factors on bone mass later in life." Osteoporosis Int.
    1993; 22:684–691

"The Mercury Story." Pbs.org. Jan. 21, 2005; accessed Apr. 6, 2007,
    http://pbs.org/now/science/mercuryinfish.html

McDougall, John A., M.D. *The McDougal Program for Women: What Every Woman Needs to Know to Be Healthy for Life*. New York: A Plume Book. Published by The Penguin Group, 1999

"Milgram Experiment." Wikipedia.org, last modified Sept. 8, 2007; accessed Sept. 9, 2007, http://en.wikipedia.org/wiki/Milgram_experiment

Mills, Dixie J. MD, FACS. "Health benefits of soy—why the controversy?" Womentowomen.com, Last modified Mar. 9, 2007; accessed Mar. 21, 2007, http://www.womentowomen.com/nutritionandweightloss/healthbenefits ofsoy.asp

Moyer-Mileur, Laurie, PhD, RD. "Food cravings and what they mean." Babycenter.com. Last updated Mar 2003; accessed May 9, 2007, http://www.babycenter.com/0_food=cravings-and-what-they-mean_1313971.bc

Murray, Rich. "How Aspartame Became Legal—The Timeline." Quantumbalancing.com, Dec. 24, 2002; accessed Mar. 5, 2005, http://www.quantumbalancing.com/news/aspartameapproved.htm

Mussalli, George, MD. "Gestational Diabetes." Babycenter.com; accessed Dec. 8, 2006, http://www.babycenter.com/refcap/pregnancy/pregcomplications/2058.html

Mussallini, George, MD, and Ann Linden, CNM. "Preeclampsia." Babycenter.com, March 2007; accessed Sept. 14, 2007, http://www.babycenter.com/O_preeclampsia_257.bc

"Natural Sweeteners." Livrite.com; accessed Feb. 2, 2005, http://www.livrite.com/sweeten.htm

Neiva et al, J Pediatr (Rio J) 2003;79(1):07–12

North, K., MSc, Jean Golding, PhD., THE ALSPAC STUDY TEAM (2000). "A maternal vegetarian diet in pregnancy is associated with hypospadias." *British Journal Urology International* 85 (1), 107–113. Doi:10.1046/j.1464–410x.2000.00436.x

"Nutrition During Pregnancy for Vegetarians." Clevelandclinic.org, accessed
    Feb. 24, 2007, http://www.clevelandclinic.org/ health/health-
    info/docs/1600/1674.asp?index=4724

"Nutrition Requirements during Pregnancy." Centerforwomenshealth.com;
    accessed Jan. 30, 2007, http://www.centerforwomenshealth.com/
    pregnancy.htm

Nutt, Amy Ellis. "In the Soil, Water, Food, Air." *The [Newark] Star Ledger*,
    Dec. 8, 2000

"Obesity During Pregnancy." Pregnancy-info.net; accessed May 11, 2007,
    http://www.pregnancy-info.net/obesity_pregnancy.html

Oglesby, Christy. "Postpartum depression: More than 'baby blues'." CNN.com,
    Jun. 27, 2001; accessed Sept 10. 2007, http://archives.cnn.com/2001/
    HEALTH/parenting/06/26/postpartum.depression/

Osborne, Sally Eauclaire. "Does Soy Have a Dark Side?" Natural Health,
    March 1999; accessed Sept. 9, 2007,
    http://findarticles.com/p/articles/mi_m0NAH/is_2_29/ai_53929987

Oski, Frank A., MD. "Don't Drink Your Milk." Teach Services, Inc. Brushton,
    NY: 1996.

Osterweil, Neil. "Filthy Lucre." Webmd.com, May 23, 2001; accessed Sept. 9,
    2007, http://www.webmd.com/news/20010523/filthy-lucre

Parpia Khan, Sheri Lyn. "Maternal Nutrition during Breastfeeding."
    Lalecheleague.org. From *New Beginnings*, Vol. 21 No. 2 March–April 2004,
    p.44; accessed May 18, 2007, http://www.lalecheleague.org/NB/
    NBMarApr04p44.html

"Pesticides Raise Child Risk of Leukemia-Study." Organicconsumers.org.
    Jan. 17, 2006; accessed Sept. 9, 2007,
    http://www.organicconsumers.org/school/leukaemia012006.cfm

Pisacane, A. "Breast-feeding and inguinal hernia." Journal of Pediatrics 1995: Vol 127, No. 1, pp 109-111

"Postpartum Bleeding." Epigee.org; accessed Sept 10, 2007, http://www.epigee.org/fetal/post_bleeding.html

"Postpartum Depression." Med.umich.edu; accessed Sept. 14, 2007, http://www.med.umich.edu/1libr/wha/wha_postpart_bha.htm

"Postpartum Depression: Symptoms, Treatment, and Support." Helpguide.org. Last modified Jan. 21, 2007; accessed Sept 10. 2007, http://www.helpguide.org/mental/postpartum_depression.htm

"Pregnancy and Constipation." Americanpregnancy.org; accessed Mar. 21, 2007, http://www.americanpregnancy.org/pregnancyhealth/constipation.html

"Pregnancy Food Cravings: What Pregnant Women Crave and Why." Epigee.org; accessed May 10, 2007, http://www.epigee.org/pregnant_diet.html

"Pregnancy & Nutrition." Womenshealthchannel.com; accessed May 11, 2007, http://www.womenshealthchannel.com/nutrition

"Pregnant women, avoid eating undercooked meat: study." Cbc.ca, Nov. 10, 2000; accessed on Mar. 2, 2007, http://www.cbc.ca/news/story/2000/07/14/toxoplasmosis000714.html

"Pregnancy and Weight Gain: How Much Is Too Much?" Epigee.org; accessed May 11, 2007, http://www.epigee.org/pregnancy/weight.html

Pritzker, Ruohonen. "Listeria Recall: Wal-Mart Egg Salad." Pritzkerlaw.com. Oct. 17, 2006; accessed Mar. 13, 2007, http://foodpoisoning.pritzkerlaw.com/archives/listeria-listeria-recall-wal-mart-egg-salad.html

"Protein: Moving Closer to Center Stage." Harvard.edu; accessed Mar. 13, 2007, http://www.hsph.harvard.edu/nutritionsource/protein.html

Quaid, Libby. Associated Press. "Government Refusal to let Kansas Meatpacker Test Cows For Mad Cow Disease Spars Lawsuit." Organicconsumers.org, Mar. 22, 2006; accessed Sept. 9, 2007, http://www.organicconsumers.org/madcow/lawsuit060326.cfm

Raffelock, Dean, DC, Dipl. Ac., CCN, Robert Roundtree, MD and Virginia Hopkins with Melissa Block. *A Natural Guide to Pregnancy and Postpartum Health*. New York: Avery, a member of Penguin Putnam, Inc., New York: 2002

Rauch, Molly. "Animal products in pregnancy." Findarticles.com. May–June 2004; accessed Feb. 12, 2007, http://www.findarticles.com/p/articles/mi_m0838/is_124/ai_n6023925

"rBGH to Blame for Rise in Twin Birth?" Organicconsumers.org. May 22, 2006; accessed Feb. 9, 2007, http://organicconsumers.org/articles/article_512.cfm

"Recalls and Field Corrections: Foods Class I." Enforcement report. FDA.gov, Feb. 5, 2003; accessed Sept. 9, 2007, http://www.fda.gov/bbs/topics/enforce/2003/ENF00781.html

"Recalls and Field Corrections: Foods Class II." Enforcement report. FDA.gov, Sept. 6, 2000; accessed Sept. 9, 2007, http://www.fda.gov/bbs/topics/ENFORCE/ENF00658.html

Rich, Deborah K. "Organic fruits and vegetables work harder for their nutrients. Produce has been losing vitamins and minerals over the past half-century." San Francisco Chronicle. Sfgate.com.Mar. 25, 2006; accessed Mar. 13, 2007, http://www.sfgate.com/cgi-bin/article.cgi?f=/c/a/2006/03/25/HOG3BHSDPG1.DTL

"The Right Formula? Soymilk vs. Cow's Milk." Webmd. Last review Jan. 30, 2005; accessed Sept. 9, 2007, http://www.medicinenet.com/script/main/art.asp?articlekey=51615

Riley, Laura, MD, OB/GYN and Stacey Nelson, MS, RD, LDN. *You and Your Baby: Healthy Eating During Pregnancy. Your Guide to Eating Well and Staying Fit*. Iowa: Meredith Books, 2006

Robbins, John. *Diet for a New America*. Walpole, NH: Stillpoint, 1987.

Robbins, John. "What About Soy?" Foodrevolution.org; accessed Mar. 1, 2007, http://www.foodrevolution.org/what_about_soy.htm

Roberts, H. J, MD., FACP, FCCP. "Aspartame Disease: An FDA-Approved Epidemic." Jan 2004; accessed Jan. 24, 2007, http://www.mercola.com/2004/jan/7/aspartame_disease.htm

Roberts, Dr. Holly, DO, FACOG. *Your Vegetarian Pregnancy: A Month by Month Guide to Health and Nutrition*. New York: A Fireside Book. Published by Simon & Schuster, 2003

Rodriguez, Lisa, RN, and Marjorie Greenfield, MD. "Vaginal Bleeding After Delivery." Drspock.com. Reviewed and revised on Aug. 25, 2004; accessed Sept. 10, 2007, http://www.drspock.com/article/0,1510,5246,00.html

Romm, Aviva Jill. The Natural Pregnancy Book. *Herbs, Nutrition, and Other Holistic Choices*. Berkeley/Toronto: Celestial Arts, 2003

Rosenblatt, KA et al "Prolonged lactation and endometrial cancer." Int. J. Epidemiol. 1995; 24:499–503

Ross-Flanigan, Nancy. "A link between sugar and heart defects." Yale.edu. Summer 2003; accessed Jan. 24, 2007, http://yalemedicine.yale.edu/ym_su03/findings.html

Ross, Jill. "Mom's Weight Can Be Big Risk for Baby." Healthatoz.com. Reviewed June 2006; accessed May 11, 2007, http://www.healthatoz.com/healthatoz/Atoz/common/standard/transform.jsp?requestURI=/healthatoz/Atoz/hc/wom/preg/alert04032002.jsp

"Salmon farms producing tainted fish-farmed salmon not as healthy as wild salmon and fish farming industry pollutes the ocean." *New York Times*. May 28, 2003; accessed Sept. 9, 2007, http://www.findarticles.com/p/articles/mi_m0876/is_86/ai_111303246

Saxe, Gordon M.D., Ph.D. "Ask the Doctor." *The Cancer Project News*, Summer 2006; accessed Dec. 5, 2007, www.cancerproject.org/media/newsletter/jul06/ask.php

Schlosser, Eric. The Cow Jumped Over the U.S.D.A." *New York Times*, Jan. 2, 2004; accessed Mar. 1, 2005, http://www.commondreams.org/views04/0102-06.htm

Schmidt, Charles W. "Poisoning Young Minds." Mindfully.org. Environmental Health Perspectives V.107, N.6, Jun 99; accessed Mar. 6, 2007, http://www.mindfully.org/Pesticide/Poisoning-Minds.htm

Schuler, Kathleen. "Smart Meat and Dairy Guide for Parents and Children." IATP.ORG; accessed Mar. 10, 2007, http://www.healthobservatory.org/library.cfm?RefID=72846

Sears, William, MD. "Ask Dr. Sears: Soda: Just Say No." Parenting.com. Oct 2003; accessed Sept. 12, 2007, http://www.parenting.com/parenting/pregnancy/article/0,19840,648325,00.html

Sears, William, MD. "Midwiferytoday Forums." Midwiferytoday.com; accessed Sept. 14, 2007; http://www.midwiferytoday.com/forums/topic.asp?TOPIC_ID=7387

"The Secret Dangers of Splenda (Sucralose), an Artificial Sweetener." Mercola.com; accessed Sept. 14, 2007, http://www.mercola.com/2000/dec/3/sucralose_dangers.htm

"75 Percent of Women Indulge Food Cravings During Pregnancy; Only 8 Percent Reach for Healthy Substitutes." Abbott.com. Apr. 4, 2005; accessed May 10, 2007, http://www.abbott.com/global/url/pressRelease/en_US/60.5:5/Press_Release_0031.htm

Sherman, Janette D., MD, *Life's Delicate Balance*, Taylor & Francis, NY, 2000

Sherman, Marjorie. "Who you calling fat? Child obesity epidemic well known, but what about those adorable bigger babies?" *The Eagle-Tribune*, Sept. 11, 2006; accessed May 18, 2007, http://babybootcamp.com/pages/news_detail.aspx?nid=82

"The Signs and Symptoms of Early Pregnancy." Mayoclinic.com; accessed Sept. 13, 2007, http://answers.yahoo.com/question/index?qid=20060824185820AAqmvMC

"Silent Spring II." Thirdworldtraveler.com. From the Summer 1997 *Food First Newsletter*; accessed Mar. 6, 2007, http://www.thirdworldtraveler.com/Environment/Silent_Spring2.html

Simontacchi, Carol. *The Crazy Makers. How the Food Industry Is Destroying Our Brains and Harming Our Children*. New York: Jeremy P. Tarcher/Putnam. A member of Penguin Putnam, Inc, 2000

"Sleep During Pregnancy." Kidshealth.org. July 2004; accessed Nov. 15, 2006, http://www.kidshealth.org/parent/pregnancy_newborn/pregnancy/sleep_during_pregnancy.html

Snuggs, Carla. "Exercise and Pregnancy." Suite101.com, Mar 16, 2007; accessed May 1, 2007, http://pregnancychildbirth.suite101.com/article.cfm/exercise_and_pregnancy

Somer, Elizabeth, M.A., R.D. *Nutrition for a Healthy Pregnancy: The Complete Guide to Eating, Before, During, and After Your Pregnancy.* Second Edition. New York: An Owl Book, Henryholt and Co, 2002.

Spock, Benjamin, MD, and Steven J. Parker, MD. *Dr. Spock's Baby and Child Care*: 7th Edition. New York: Pocket Books, a division of Simon and Schuster, 1998

Squires, Sally. "Mothers Again Urged to Eat Fish." Washingtonpost.com, Oct. 4, 2007; accessed Dec. 5, 2007, http://www.washingtonpost.com/wpdyn/content/article/2007/10/03/AR2007100301278.html?sid=ST2007102200863

"Stage by Stage, an Ingredient List for all Heinz Baby Food." Heinzbaby.com; accessed Sept. 12, 2007, http://www.heinzbaby.com/english/ingredient

Stallone, Daryth D., PhD, MPH, and Michael F. Jacobson, PhD. "Cheating Babies: Nutritional Quality and Cost of Commercial Baby Food." CSPI Reports, accessed Sept. 12, 2007, http://www.cspinet.org/reports/cheat1.html

"Statement of H. J. Roberts, MD., Concerning the Use of Products Containing Aspartame (nutrasweet) by Persons with Diabetes and hypoglycemia." Geocities.com, accessed Sept. 10, 2007, http://www.geocities.com/hotsprings/4578/page9.html

Strom, Brian L., MD; Rita Schinnar, MPA; Echard E. Zeigler, MD; Kurt T. Barnhart, MD; Mary D. Sammuel, ScD; George A. Macones, MD; Virginia A. Stallings, MD; Jean M. Drulis, BA; Steven E. Nelson, BA; Sandra A. Hanson, BA. "Exposure to Soy-Based Formula in Infancy and Endocrinological and Reproductive Outcomes in Young Adulthood." *Journal of the American Medical Association*. Vol. 286 No. 7, 807–814. Aug. 15, 2001; accessed Sept. 8, 2007, http://jama.ama-assn.org/cgi/content/full/ 286/7/807

"Study: Pesticide May Reduce Fertility." Organicconsumers.org, published Jan. 12, 2006; accessed Sept. 9, 2007, http://www.organicconsumers.org/toxic/testosterone011706.cfm

"Sugar Blues." Natural Nutrition; accessed Feb. 2, 2005, http://livrite.com/sugar1.htm

"10 Reasons to Avoid Acidosis." PolyMVASurvivors.com; accessed Mar. 28, 2005, http://polymvasurvivors.com/4corners_coral.html

"¾ Chickens Bought Nationwide Harbor Salmonella or Campylobacter." Organicconsumers.org. Consumer Reports Jan 2003; accessed Mar. 13, 2007, http://www.organicconsumers.org/toxic/chixyuck.cfm

"Top 10 Reasons Not to Eat Chickens." Goveg.com; accessed Mar. 13, 2007, http://www.goveg.com/f-top10chickens.asp

"ToxFAQs for Methylene Chloride." Agency for Toxic Substances & Disease Registry; accessed Sept. 13, 2007, http://www.atsdr.cdc.gov/tfacts14.html

"Toxic Shock." Goveg.com; accessed Mar. 13, 2007, http://goveg.com/contamination.asp

Turner, Dr. Natasha, ND. "The Perils of Sugar." Truestarhealth.com; accessed Jan. 24, 2007, http://www.truestarhealth.com/members/archives.asp?content=14ml3pla95

"Understanding Food Cravings." Drbriffa.com. Nov. 7, 2000; accessed May 9, 2007, http://www.drbriffa.com/blog/2000/11/07/understanding-food-cravings

"Union of Concerned Scientists Food & Farming Newsletter." Organicconsumers.org, April 2006; accessed Sept. 9, 2007, http://organic-consumers.org/politics/FEED060417.cfm

"Unsafe and Unethical. FDA Poised to Approve Cloned Animals for Consumption." *Farm Sanctuary News*. Spring 2007: 18

"USDA Attempts to Pack Organic Standards Board with Corporate Agribusiness Reps: Organic Consumers Fight Hijacked Seats on NOSB." Organic Consumers Association, Dec. 7, 2006; accessed Sept. 9, 2007, http://www.organicconsumers.org/articles/article_3526.cfm

"USDA Cover-Up of Mad Cow Cases." Organicconsumers.org, May 10, 2005; accessed Jun. 1, 2005, http://www.organicconsumers.org/bytes/051005.cfm

"USDA looking to allow yet more synthetic chemicals in organic meat." Newstarget.com. Originally published Jul. 21, 2006; accessed Feb. 28, 2007, http://www.newstarget.com/z019727.html

"USDA Orders Recall of 143 Million Pounds of Beef." CNN.com, February 18, 2008; accessed March 6, 2008, http://www.cnn.com/2008/HEALTH/02/17/beef.recall/

U.S. Department of Health and Human Services. "Symptoms Attributed to Aspartame in Complaints Submitted to the FDA." Apr. 20, 1995; accessed Feb. 22, 2005, http://www.presidiotex.com/aspartame/Facts/92_Symptoms/92_symptoms.html

"U.S. Government Facts: Children's Chemical & Pesticide Exposure via Food Products." Organicconsumers.org; accessed Mar 2007, http://www.organic-consumers.org/organic/wic-faq.pdf

"USTR demands Japan lift beef import restrictions linked to cow age." Japan Today online, accessed Sept. 15, 2007, http://www.japantoday.com/jp/news/400520

"Veg 101 FAQ." Vegetariantimes.com; accessed Feb. 24, 2007,
  http://www.vegetariantimes.com/section_display.cfm?section_id=92

"Vegetarian Diets for Children: Right from the Start." Pcrm.org; accessed Sept.
  9, 2007, http://www.pcrm.org/health.veginfo/veg_diets_for_children.html

"Vegetarian diets for pregnancy and children." Peta.org.uk; accessed Dec. 6,
  2006, http://www.peta.org.uk/feat/UKvegkit/pregnancy.asp

Vincent, Beth, MHS. "The importance of DHA during pregnancy and
  breastfeeding." Pregnancyandbaby.com; accessed Sept. 9, 2007,
  http://pregnancyandbaby.com/pregnancy/baby/The-importance-of-DHA-
  during-pregnancy-and-breastfeeding-5726.htm

"Vitamins and Minerals. What You Eat is Just as Important as How Much You
  Eat." Pregnancy-info.net; accessed Sept. 12, 2007, http://www.pregnancy-
  info.net/vitamins.html

Waldman, Peter. "Ingredients in cosmetics, toys a safety concern." *The Wall
  Street Journal* BC-WSJ-toxic traces, 2853. Tues. Oct. 4, 2005; accessed Sept 9.
  2007, http://www.post-gazette.com/pg/05277/582410.stm

Wangen, Stephen N.D. "Food Allergy Solutions Review."
  FoodAllergySolutions.com, July 2003; accessed March 28, 2005,
  http://www.foodallergysolutions.com/food-allergy-news0307.html

Warren, Beth. "Vegan parents guilty in infant murder—6 week old starved to
  death fed diet of soymilk & apple juice." AJC Online (*Atlanta Journal-
  Constitution*) Published May 2, 2007; accessed June 12, 2007,
  http://www.ajc.com/metro/content/metro/atlanta/stories/2007/05/02/
  0502vegans.html

Washam, Cynthia. "Concentrating on PBDEs. Chemical Levels Rise in
  Women." Ehponline.org; accessed Feb. 12, 2007,
  http://www.ehponline.org/docs/2003/111-9/ss.html

Washam, Cynthia. "Suspect Inheritance. Potential Neurotoxicants Passed to

Fetuses." Volume 111, Number 9. Ehponline.org. July 2003; accessed Feb. 12, 2007, http://www.ehponline.org/docs/2003/111-9/ss.html

Watkins, Lucy p. "Dealing with Dairy Allergies in Your Nursling." Vegetarianbaby.com; accessed Nov. 30, 2006, http://vegetarianbaby.com/articles/dairyallergies.shtml

Weed, Susan S. *Wise Woman Herbal for the Childbearing Year*. Woodstock, New York: Ash Tree Publishing, 1986.

"Weight gain during pregnancy." Health24.com; accessed Sept. 7, 2007, http://www.health24.com/dietnfood/DietDocs_articles/15-1871,22918.asp

"What is gestational diabetes?" Bupa.co.uk. August 2003; accessed Nov 2006, http://hcd2/bupa.co.uk/fact_sheets/html/diabetes_in_pregnancy.html

"What Precautions Should I Take When I Am Pregnant or Nursing?" Drfuhrman.com; accessed Nov. 21, 2006, http://www.drfuhrman.com/disease/pregnancy.aspx

"What's Wrong with Dairy Products?" Pcrm.org; accessed Feb. 13, 2007, http://www.pcrm.org/health/veginfo/dairy.html

"What You Eat Is Just as Important as How Much You Eat." Pregnancyinfo.net; accessed May 12, 2007, http://www.pregnancy-info.net/vitamins

"What You Should Know About Chemicals in Your Cosmetics." *Consumer Reports*. Winter 2007; accessed Sept. 10, 2007, http://www.safecosmetics.org/newsroom/consumer_repts_1_07.cfm

"When do most couples start having sex again after their baby is born?" Babycenter.com; accessed Sept 10. 2007, http://www.babycenter.com/expert/baby/postpartumsex/11805.html

"Which foods should I avoid during pregnancy?" nhsdirect.nhs.uk, accessed on Nov. 21, 2006, http://www.nhsdirect.nhs.uk/articles/article.aspx?articleId=917

Whitney, Eleanor Noss, and Sharon Rady Rolfes. *Understanding Nutrition*, 8th ed. Belmont: Wadsworth, 1999

"Why Animal Agriculture Doesn't Add Up." Goveg.com, accessed Dec. 5, 2007, http://www.goveg.com/worldHunger-animalAgriculture.asp

"Why Exercise During Pregnancy?" Womenshealth.gov. Mar 2007; accessed May 18, 2007, http://www.womenshealth.gov/pregnancy/pregnancy/fit.cfm

Williams, Rose Marie. "'What's in the Beef?'(Interview with Howard Lyman, author of *Mad Cowboy*.) (Discussion of health aspects of additives in beef)." Encyclopedia.com. Oct. 1, 2001; accessed Mar. 6, 2007, http://www.encyclopedia.com/doc/1G1-78900860.html

Williams, R.M., TLfDP #203, pp 26, 27 (an endnote)

Wilson, Melanie. "A Successful Veg Pregnancy." Vegetarianbaby.com; accessed Nov. 21, 2006, http://www.vegetarianbaby.com/articles/successpreg.shtml

"Wise Use of Herbs and Vitamins During Pregnancy." Childbirthsolutions.com; accessed June 26, 2006, http://www.childbirthsolutions.com/articles/pregnancy/herbsandvit/index.php

Woolston, Chris. "Artificial Sweeteners and Pregnancy." Ahealthyme.com; accessed Sept. 14, 2007, http://www.ahealthyme.com/topic/sweeteners

Yntema, Sharon. Vegetarian Pregnancy. *The definitive nutritional Guide to Having a Healthy Baby*. Ithaca, New York: McBooks Press, 1994.

Young, Robert O., Ph.D., and Shelley Redford Young. *The pH Miracle: Balance Your Diet, Reclaim Your Health*. New York: Warner, 2002

Zeretzke, Karen. "Allergies and the Breastfeeding Family." *New Beginnings*. Vol. 15 no.4 Jul-Aug 1998 p.100; accessed Sept. 9, 2007, http://www.lalecheleague.org/NB/NBJulAug98p100.html

Notes

[1] Lauersen and Bouchez, *Getting Pregnant: What You Need to Know Right Now*, 334.

[2] Ibid., 335.

[3] Eisenberg, Hathaway, and Murkoff, *What to Expect When You're Expecting*, 53.

[4] Plumbo, "Is an occasional glass of wine okay?" ivillage.com.

[5] "Birth Defect Statistics," pcrm.org.

[6] Eisenberg, Hathaway, and Murkoff, 60.

[7] Ibid., 60.

[8] "Caffeine," ucheepines.org.

[9] Curtis and Schuler, *Your Pregnancy Week by Week*, 62.

[10] Eisenberg, Hathaway, and Murkoff, 53.

[11] *Caffeine Facts*, shapefit.com.

[12] Eisenberg, Hathaway, and Murkoff, 60.

[13] Ibid.

[14] "ToxFAQs for Methylene Chloride," atsdr.cdc.gov.

[15] Sears, parenting.com.

[16] Maugh, "Diet soda, metabolic syndrome linked," LAtimes.com.

[17] "Aspartame: What you Don't Know Can Hurt You," mercola.com.

[18] Somer, *Nutrition for a Healthy Pregnancy*, 203.

[19] "Birth Defects," clevelandclinic.org.

[20] "Over-the-counter medicines in pregnancy," netdoctor.co.uk.

[21] "Birth Defects and Pharmaceutical Drugs," oshmanlaw.com.

[22] "Over-the-counter medicines in pregnancy," netdoctor.co.uk.

[23] Ibid.

[24] Curtis and Schuler, *Your Pregnancy Week by Week*, 88.

[25] Ibid.

[26] "Back pain during pregnancy," mayoclinic.com.

[27] Ibid.

[28] "Causes of Shortness of Breath During Pregnancy," marchofdimes.com.

[29] "The Signs and Symptoms of Early Pregnancy," mayoclinic.com.

[30] Burch and Sachs, *Natural Healing for the Pregnant Woman*, 139–141.

[31] Ibid., 149.

[32] Somer, 153.

[33] Ibid., 179.

[34] Ibid., 126–127.

[35] Beck, *The Ultimate Nutrition Guide for Women*, 270–271.

[36] Greenfield, "Vaginal Infections during Pregnancy" drspock.com.

[37] Linden, "Vaginal discharge during pregnancy," babycenter.com.

[38] "Sleeping During Pregnancy," kidshealth.org.

[40] Turner, "The Perils of Sugar," truestarhealth.com.

[41] Chandel, "Sweet poison," The Sunday Tribune Spectrum, tribuneindia.com.

[42] Somer, 143.

[43] Johnson, "High Sugar, Fat Intake During Early Pregnancy Increases Preeclampsia Risk," findarticles.com.

[44] Turner, "The Perils of Sugar," truestarhealth.com.

[45] "Gestational Diabetes: Causes, Symptoms and Management," womenfitness.net.

[46] Mussalli, "Gestational Diabetes," babycenter.com.

[47] Ibid.

[48] Ibid.

[49] Ibid.

[50] Manzella, "A Fiber-Rich Diet Decreases Risk for Gestational Diabetes," diabetes.org.uk.

[51] Ross-Flanigan, "A link between sugar and heart defects," yalemedicine.yale.edu.

[52] Mussalli, "Gestational Diabetes," babycenter.com.

[53] Ibid.

[54] Turner, truestarhealth.com.

[55] "Sugar Blues," liverite.com.

[56] Sears, "Midwifery Forums," midwiferytoday.com.

[57] Woolston, "Artificial Sweeteners and Pregnancy," ahealthyme.com.

[58] "Food Additives/Preservatives and Pregnancy," pregnancyweekly.com.

[59] Department of Health and Human Services-Symptoms Attributed to Aspartame in Complaints Submitted to the FDA," U.S. Department of Health and Human Services, presidiotex.com.

[60] Roberts, "Aspartame Disease: An FDA-Approved Epidemic," mercola.com.

[61] Gold, "Common Toxic and Substances to Avoid," holisiticmed.com.

[62] "Aspartame: What You Don't Know Can Hurt You," mercola.com.

[63] Murray, "How Aspartame Became Legal—The Timeline," quantumbalancing.com.

[64] Ibid.

[65] Ibid.

[66] Ibid.

[67] "Aspartame: What You Don't Know Can Hurt You," mercola.com.

[68] Johnson, "Aspartame . . . a Killer!" *The Sunday Express London*, newfrontier.com.

[69] Martini, "Report for Schools, OB-GYN and Pediatricians on Children and Aspartame/MSG," wnho.net.

[70] Gold, "Formaldehyde Poisoning from Aspartame," holisticmed.com.

[71] Martini, Wnho.net.

[72] Ibid.

[73] "Statement of H.J Roberts. M.D., Concerning the Use of Products Containing Aspartame (NutraSweet) by Persons with Diabetes and hypoglycemia." geocities.com.

[74] Roberts, "Aspartame Disease: An FDA-Approved Epdemic," mercola.com.

[75] Martini, Wnho.net.

[76] Ibid.

[77] "Aspartame What You Don't Know Can Hurt You. Natural Ingredients Imply 'Not Harmful,'" mercola.com.

[78] Ibid.

[79] Mercola, "The Secret Dangers of Splenda (Sucralose). An Artificial Sweetener," mercola.com.

[80] Ibid.

[81] Ibid.

[82] Ibid.

[83] Ibid.

[84] Ibid.

[85] Ibid.

[86] Ibid.

[87] Young, *The pH Miracle: Balance Your Diet, Reclaim Your Health*, 50–51.

[88] Ibid., 14–15.

[89] "10 Reasons to Avoid Acidosis," polymvasurvivors.com.

[90] Young, 24–25.

[91] Young, 51–52.

[92] "Natural Sweeteners, Natural Nutrition," liverite.com.

[93] Whitney and Rolfes, *Understanding Nutrition*, 44.

[94] Riley and Nelson, *You and Your Baby*, 38.

[95] Somer, 70.

[96] Ibid., 179.

[97] "Nutrition Requirements during Pregnancy," Centerforwomenshealth.com.

[98] Desjardins, "Just Say No to a Low Carbohydrate Diet," todaysparent.com.

[99] Durocher, "The Low-Carb Craze. Should Pregnant Women Participate?" pregnancytoday.com.

[100] Somer, 28.

[101] "Milgram Experiment," wikipedia.org.

[102] "What's Wrong with Dairy Products?" pcrm.org

[103] Campbell and Campbell II, *The China Study,* 205.

[104] Ibid., 204.

[105] Robbins, *Diet for a New America*, 164.

106 Watkins, "Dealing with Dairy Allergies in Your Nursling," vegetarianbaby.com.

107 Roberts, *Your Vegetarian Pregnancy.* 172

108 Ibid., 230.

109 "What's Wrong with Dairy Products?" pcrm.org.

110 Campbell and Campbell II, xv–368.

111 Ibid., 6.

112 Ibid., 49–50.

113 Ibid., 6.

114 Robbins, *Diet for a New America*, 150.

115 Campbell and Campbell II, 292.

116 "What's Wrong with Dairy Products?" pcrm.org.

117 Cousens, *Conscious Eating*, 73.

118 Benjamin and Parker, *Dr. Spock's Baby and Child Care*, 341.

119 Wangen, "Food Allergy Solutions Review," foodallergysolutions.com.

120 Kradjian, "The Milk Letter: A Message to My Patients," vegsource.com.

121 Holford, *The Optimum Nutrition Bible*, 43.

122 "What's Wrong with Dairy Products?" pcrm.org.

123 Oski, *Don't Drink Your Milk*, 12.

124 Kradjian, vegsource.com.

125 Epstein, *What's in Your Milk?* xxvi–xxvii.

126 Ibid., xxiii.

127 Ibid.

128 Ibid.

[129] Ibid., 34.

[130] Ibid.

[131] Donohoe, "Letter to the Editor of Wall Street Journal—Long Standing Evidence of rBGH Dangers," organicconsumers.org.

[132] Ibid., 7.

[133] Kradjian, vegsource.com.

[134] Gelles, "Why Antibiotics in Meat Should Give You Pause," *The Philadelphia Inquirer.*

[135] Epstein, 34–35.

[136] "rBGH to Blame for Rise in Twin Birth?" organicconsumers.org.

[137] Donohoe, organicconsumers.org.

[138] Green, "Not Milk: The USDA, Monsanto, and the U.S. Dairy Industry," LiPMagazine.

[139] Kradjian, vegsource.com.

[140] Cousens, 478.

[141] Rauch, "Animal products in pregnancy," findarticles.com.

[142] Schuler, "Smart Meat and Dairy Guide for Parents and Children," iatp.org.

[143] Ibid.

[144] Ibid.

[145] Washam, "Suspect Inheritance. Potential Neurotoxicants Passed to Fetuses," ehponline.org.

[146] Steinman, *Diet for a Poisoned Planet*, 122.

[147] Greger, "Paratuberculosis and Crohn's Disease: Got Milk?" veganoutreach.org.

[148] Kradjian, vegsource.com.

[149] Ibid.

[150] "Low-Fat Dairy Products Linked to Increased Infertility Risk," pcrm.org.

[151] Kradjian, vegsource.com.

[152] Cousens, 479.

[153] Campbell and Campbell II, xv–368.

[154] "What's Wrong with Dairy Products?" pcrm.org.

[155] Roberts, 173.

[156] Riley, 33 and McDougall, *The McDougal Program for Women*, 50.

[157] Holford, 42.

[158] Riley, 91.

[159] Romm, *The Natural Pregnancy Book*, 71.

[160] Roberts, 110.

[161] Romm, 225.

[162] Roberts, 235.

[163] Wilson, "A Successful Veg Pregnancy," vegetarianbaby.com

[164] Roberts, 69.

[165] "Protein: Moving Closer to Center Stage," hsph.Harvard.edu.

[166] Gates, "The Surprising Reason You May Be Aging Prematurely Improper Protein Digestion," bodyecology.com.

[167] Chavarro, Willett, and Skerrett, "Fat, Carbs, and the Science of Conception," Newsweek.

[168] "Animal protein & fat raise endometrial cancer," reuters.com, International Journal of Cancer, reuters.com.

[169] Herrick, Phillips, Haselden, Shiell, Campbell-Brown and Godfrey. "Maternal Consumption of a High-Meat, Low-Carbohydrate Diet in Late Pregnancy: Relation to Adult Cortisol Concentrations in the

Offspring." The Journal of Clinical Endocrinology & Metabolism, Jcem.org.

[170] Meldung, "High protein/low carbohydrate diet when pregnant leads to higher stress susceptibility in children." Innovations-report.de.

[171] "What's Wrong with Dairy Products?" pcrm.org.

[172] "Full Profile. Nitrite, Nitrate," checnet.org.

[173] "Hormone Replacement Increases Cancer Risk." Good Medicine Magazine, pcrm.org

[174] Saxe, "Ask the Doctor," cancerproject.org.

[175] "Toxic Shock," goveg.com and Nutt, "In the Soil, Water, Food, Air," The [Newark] Star-Ledger.

[176] "Pregnant women, avoid eating undercooked meat—study," cbc.ca.

[177] Andersson, "Food-Borne Risks in Pregnancy," willystreet.coop.

[178] Pritzker, "Listeria Recall: Wal-Mart Egg Salad," foodpoisoning.pritzkerlaw.com.

[179] "3/4 Chickens Bought Nationwide Harbor Salmonella or Campylobacter," organicconsumers.org.

[180] "Eggs Non Gratis," The Civil Abolitionist, weblinknn.com.

[181] "Top 10 Reasons Not to Eat Chickens,"goveg.com.

[182] "E. Coli Infection." American Academy of Family Physicians, Familydoctor.org.

[183] "¾ Chickens Bought Nationwide Harbor Salmonella or Campylobacter," organicconsumers.org.

[184] Freedman and Barnouin, *Skinny Bitch*, 44–45.

[185] Gelles, "Why Antibiotics in Meat Should Give You Pause," *The Philadelphia Inquirer*.

[186] "Drug-Resistant Bacteria Found in U.S. Meat," Reuters Medical News, 24 May 2001.

[187] Williams, "'What's in the Beef?' Interview with Howard Lyman, author of *Mad Cowboy*. Discussion of health aspects of additives in beef," Encyclopedia.com. and Williams, R.M., TLfDP #203, 26–27 (endnote).

[188] "Union of Concerned Scientists Food & Farming Newsletter," organicconsumers.org.

[189] Roberts, 169.

[190] Williams, "What's in the Beef?" and Epstein, *The Politics of Cancer*, encyclopedia.com.

[191] Williams, "What's in the Beef?" and Sherman, *Life's Delicate Balance*, encyclopedia.com.

[192] Williams, "What's in the Beef?" and Epstein, *The Politics of Cancer*, encyclopedia.com.

[193] Williams, "What's in the Beef?" and Epstein, *The Politics of Cancer*, encyclopedia.com.

[194] Holford, 40.

[195] Freni-Titulaer, Cordero, Haddock, Lebron, Martinez, and Mills, "Premature Thelarche in Puerto Rico. A Search for Environmental Factors," American Journal of Diseases of Children, 40 (1986): 1263–1267.

[196] "Meat-Eating Moms Have Less Fertile Sons," pcrm.org

[197] Gillette, "Premature Puberty: Is Early Sexual Development the Price of Pollution?" E: The Environmental Magazine.

[198] "Link Eyed Between Beef and Cancer. Tests Show Likely Link Between Growth Hormone and Breast Cancer,"cbsnews.com.

[199] Schlosser, "The Cow Jumped Over the U.S.D.A," *New York Times*, commondreams.org.

[200] Martin, Andrew, "How to Add Oomph to 'Organic,'" Nytimes.org.

[201] Coupe, "Editorial: Mad Cows, Lunatic Politicians, & The Case for Traceback," cattlenetwork.com.

[202] "USTR demands Japan lift beef import restrictions linked to cow age," Japan Today, japantoday.com.

[203] Barnard, "Meat Too Tough to Eat," Hartford Courant, pcrm.org.

[204] "Silent Spring II," thirdworldtraveler.com.

[205] Williams, Rose Marie, "'What's in the Beef?'(Interview with Howard Lyman, author of *Mad Cowboy*. Discussion of health aspects of additives in beef)," Encyclopedia.com.

[206] Roberts, 148 and 207.

[207] "A Cesspool of Pollutants. Now Is the Time to Clean-Up Your Body," nealhendrickson.com.

[208] "Silent Spring II," www.thirdworldtraveler.com.

[209] "Fetal Death and Growth Retardation," georgiastrait.org.

[210] "A Cesspool of Pollutants. Now Is the Time to Clean-Up Your Body," nealhendrickson.com.

[211] Geller, "Questions About Pesticides On Foods," Journal of Medical Toxicology.

[212] Schmidt, "Poisoning Young Minds," Environmental Health Perspectives, mindfully.org.

[213] "Silent Spring II," www.thirdworldtraveler.com.

[214] Watkins, Lucy "Dealing with Dairy Allergies in Your Nursling," vegetarianbaby.com.

[215] Squires, "Mothers Again Urged to Eat Fish," washingtonpost.com.

[216] "Fishy Advice, " VegNews, 29.

[217] Ibid.

[218] "What Precautions Should I Take When I Am Pregnant or Nursing?" drfurhman.com.

[219] "A Cesspool of Pollutants. Now Is the Time to Clean-Up Your Body," nealhendrickson.com.

[220] "Salmon farms producing tainted fish-farmed salmon not as healthy as wild salmon and fish farming industry pollutes the ocean," New York Times, findarticles.com.

[221] Hooper, "Risks and benefits of omega 3 fats for mortality, cardiovascular disease and cancer: systemic review," *British Medical Journal*, bmj.com.

[222] Ferdowsian, and Levin, "Fish Still Not a Healthy Choice," *The Providence Journal*, pcrm.org.

[223] Riley and Nelson, 90.

[224] Roberts, 67–68.

[225] Robbins, "What about Soy?" foodrevolution.org.

[226] Mills, "Health benefits of soy—why the controversy?" womentowomen.com.

[227] Roberts, 35.

[228] Mills, womentowomen.com.

[229] Roberts, 35.

[230] Robbins, "What About Soy?" foodrevolution.org.

[231] Mills, womentowomen.com.

[232] Robbins, "What About Soy?" foodrevolution.org.

[233] Mills, womentowomen.com.

[234] Osborne, Sally Eauclaire, "Does Soy Have a Dark Side?" Natural Health, findarticles.com.

[235] Elliot, "Mother and Baby Guide," viva.org.uk.

[236] Eisnitz, *Slaughterhouse*, 20.

[237] Ibid., 66.

[238] Ibid., 69–70.

[239] Ibid., 126–133.

[240] Ibid., 29.

[241] Ibid., 20, 28–29.

[242] Ibid., 71.

[243] Ibid., 166.

[244] Ibid., 166.

[245] Ibid., 166.

[246] Ibid., 166.

[247] Ibid., front jacket.

[248] Ibid., 124.

[249] Ibid., 82.

[250] Ibid., 125.

[251] Ibid., 87.

[252] Ibid., 84.

[253] Ibid., 91.

[254] Ibid., 130.

[255] Ibid., 132–133.

[256] Ibid., 144–145

[257] Ibid., 145.

[258] Ibid., 93.

[259] Ibid., 133.

[260] Ibid., 140–141.

[261] Ibid., 172.

[262] Ibid.

[263] Ibid., 173.

[264] Ibid., 174.

[265] Ibid., 175.

[266] "Free-Range Eggs and Meat: Conning Consumers?" Peta.org.

[267] "Investigation Reveals Slaughter Horrors at Agriprocessors," Peta.org.

[268] Eisnitz, 125.

[269] "USDA orders recall of 143 million pounds of beef," CNN.com.

[270] Brown, e-mail.

[271] "Animal Friendly Quotes," peta.org

[272] Grace, *A Way Out*, 8–9.

[273] Ibid., 8–10.

[274] "Veg 101 FAQ," vegetariantimes.com.

[275] Greger, "Vegan Children: A Recent Review," drgreger.org.

[276] "C-Section: Medical Reasons," marchofdimes.com.

[277] "Vegetarian diets for pregnancy and children," peta.org.uk.

[278] Ibid.

[279] "The Cost of Preeclampsia in the USA," preeclampsia.org.

[280] Greger, "Plant-Based Diets Beneficial in Pregnancy," all-creatures.org.

[281] Roberts, 20.

[282] Robbins, "What About Soy?" foodrevolution.org.

[283] Marino, "Ten Best Selling Books of All Time," Industry Week, answers.google.com.

[284] Benjamin and Parker, *Dr. Spock's Baby and Child Care*, 338–340.

[285] Warren, "Vegan parents guilty in infant murder 6 week old starved to death fed diet of soymilk & apple juice," AJC Online (*Atlanta Journal-Constitution*).

[286] North, K., Jean Golding, "A maternal vegetarian diet in pregnancy is associated with hypospadias," BJU study, 107-113.

[287] Ibid.

[288] Ibid.

[289] Golding, e-mail.

[290] "Factory Farming: Environmental Consequences," Animalalliance.ca.

[291] "Livestock a major threat to the environment," fao.org.

[292] Cook, "Environmental Hogwash," inthesetimes.com.

[293] "Why Animal Agriculture Doesn't Add Up," goveg.com.

[294] Cousens, 442.

[295] Rich, "Organic fruits and vegetables work harder for their nutrients. Produce has been losing vitamins and minerals over the past half-century," *San Francisco Chronicle*, sfgate.com.

[296] Young, 82–83.

[297] Howell, Enzyme Nutrition, 4.

[298] Howell, Enzyme Nutrition, 4–5.

[299] "Constipation," healthynj.org.

[300] "Pregnancy and Constipation," americanpregnancy.org.

[301] Levis, "Dealing with Constipation during Pregnancy," amazingpregnancy.com.

[302] "Constipation during pregnancy," health-cares.net.

[303] "Pregnancy and Constipation," americanpregnancy.org.

[304] Ibid.

[305] "Fantastic Fiber," askdrsears.com.

[306] "Constipation During Pregnancy," solutions.psu.edu.

[307] Clark, "The Athlete's Kitchen. Roughing-up Your Sports Diet," facilities.princeton.edu.

[308] "Foods Rich in Fiber," ivillage.com.

[309] "Fantastic Fiber," askdrsears.com.

[311] Roberts, 21.

[312] Roberts, 170.

[313] Manzella, "A Fiber-Rich Diet Decreases Risk for Gestational Diabetes," diabetes.about.

[314] Barnes, "Maternity Leave Helps Banish the Baby Blues," babyfit.com.

[315] "Eating Disorders during Pregnancy," americanpregnancy.org.

[316] "Is It Safe for My Baby?—Laxatives," camh.net.

[317] Cropper, "Does It Pay To Buy Organic?" businessweek.com.

[318] Fialka, "EPA Scientists Cite Pressure in Pesticide Study," Wall Street Journal Online, online.wsj.com.

[319] "EPA's Latest Human Pesticide Testing Rule Called Illegal, Immoral," ens.newswire.com.

[320] "Alert Update," organicconsumers.org.

[321] "EPA's Latest Human Pesticide Testing Rule Called Illegal, Immoral," ens.newswire.com.

[322] "Pesticides Raise Child Risk of Leukemia-Study," organicconsumers.org.

[323] "Bush EPA Nominee Abandons Insecticide-on-Children Study After Senate Hearing," wikinews.org.

[324] Kirkpatrick, "EPA Cancels Pesticide Tests On Floridian Babies," apparenting.com.

[325] "Study: Pesticide May Reduce Fertility," organicconsumers.org.

[326] "Chlorpyrifos," Wikipedia.org.

[327] "Eleven States Oppose EPA Mercury Proposal," oag.state.ny.us.

[328] "The Mercury Story," pbs.org.

[329] "Lowey Calls For Hearing on NY's Mercury Pollution As EPA Proposes Rules That Are Too Lax," house.gov.

[330] "Eleven States Oppose EPA Mercury Proposal," oag.state.ny.us.

[331] Greger, "Mercury Contamination in Fish," vegetarianbaby.com.

[332] Ibid.

[333] "USDA Cover-Up of Mad Cow Cases," Food, Consumer and Environment News—Tidbits with an Edge.

[334] Apuzzo, "Judge allows private testing for mad cow disease in U.S," organicconsumers.org.

[335] Langeland, "Tainted Meat, Tainted Money: Consumer groups decry coziness between government agribusiness," Colorado Springs Independent online.

[336] Schlosser, "The Cow Jumped Over the USDA."

[337] Quaid, "Government Refusal to let Kansas Meatpacker Test Cows For Mad Cow Disease Spars Lawsuit," organicconsumers.org.

[338] Apuzzo, organicconsumers.org.

[339] "Consumers Union & OCA Criticize USDA for Latest Appointment of So-Called Consumer Representatives to the National Organic Standards Board, organicconsumers.org.

[340] USDA Attempts to Pack Organic Standards Board with Corporate Agribusiness Reps: Organic Consumers Fight Hijacked Seats on NOSB," organicconsumers.org.

[341] "USDA looking to allow yet more synthetic chemicals in organic meat," newstarget.com.

[342] "Alert: Another Sneak Attack on Organic Standards: USDA to Allow More Conventional Ingredients in Organics," organicconsumers.org.

[343] McNeil, "U.S. Reduces Testing for Mad Cow Disease, Citing Few Infections," nytimes.com.

[344] "U.S. Government Facts: Children's Chemical & Pesticide Exposure via Food Products," organicconsumers.org.

[345] FDA's Mission Statement, U.S Food and Drug Administration, fda.gov.

[346] U.S. Government Facts: Children's Chemical & Pesticide Exposure via Food Products," organicconsumers.org.

[347] "Unsafe and Unethical. FDA Poised to Approve Cloned Animals for Consumption," Farm Sanctuary News.

[348] Schlosser, "The Cow Jumped Over the U.S.D.A." *New York Times*, commondreams.org.

[349] Barnard, *Breaking the Food Seduction*, 50–52.

[350] Ibid., 50–51.

[351] Ibid., 52.

[352] Ibid., 53.

[353] "Understanding Food Cravings," drbriffa.com.

[354] "Here's to Pickles and Ice Cream," medicinenet.com.

[355] "Pregnancy Food Cravings: What Pregnant Women Crave and Why," epigee.org.

[356] "Food cravings and what they mean," babycenter.com.

[357] Roberts, 188.

[358] Ibid., 125.

[359] Somer, 133.

[360] "Food cravings and what they mean," babycenter.com.

[361] Somer, 133.

[362] Roberts, 123.

[363] "Food cravings and what they mean," babycenter.com.

[364] Douglas, "Pregnancy Food Cravings: Fact or Fiction," pregnancyandbaby.com.

[365] Bierma, Paige. "Getting to the Bottom of Pregnancy Cravings." Healthresources.com.

[366] "Food cravings and what they mean," babycenter.com.

[367] "Understanding Food Cravings," drbriffa.com.

[368] Somer, 248.

[369] Ibid.

[370] "Food cravings and what they mean," babycenter.com.

[371] "75% of Women Indulge Food Cravings During Pregnancy, Only 8 Percent Reach For Healthy Substitutes," abbott.com.

[372] Roberts, 122.

[374] http://www.epigee.org/pregnancy/weight.html

[375] "Pregnancy & Nutrition," womenshealthchannel.com.

[376] "Eating for Two: Weight Influences on Pregnancy," Americanpregnancy.org.

[377] Artal, Catanzaro, Gavard, Mostello, and Friganza, "A lifestyle intervention of weight-gain restriction: diet and exercise in obese women with gestational diabetes mellitus," Applied Physiology, Nutrition, and Metabolism, nrc.ca.

[378] "Eating for Two: Weight Influences on Pregnancy." americanpregnancy.org.

[379] Ibid.

[380] Ibid.

[381] Ibid. and "Pregnancy and Weight Gain: How Much is Too Much?" epigee.org.

[382] "Eating for Two: Weight Influences on Pregnancy," americanpregnancy.org.

[383] Sherman, "Who you calling fat? Child obesity epidemic well known, but what about those adorable bigger babies?" The Eagle-Tribune, babybootcamp.com.

[384] "Excessive weight gain during pregnancy directly associated with having an overweight child," news-medical.net.

[385] Ross, "Mom's Weight Can Be Big Risk for Baby," healthatoz.com.

[386] Sherman, "Who you calling fat? Child obesity epidemic well known, but what about those adorable bigger babies?" The Eagle-Tribune, babybootcamp.com.

[387] "Here's essential exercise information for pregnant women, plus some gentle postpartum moves," Fit Pregnancy Magazine, August/September 2006, 124.

[388] "Why Exercise During Pregnancy?" womenshealth.gov.

[389] Snuggs, "Exercise and Pregnancy," suite101.com.

[390] Booth and Alpino, "Exercise During Pregnancy Helps You Stay Healthy," babyfit.com.

[391] "Here's essential exercise information for pregnant women, plus some gentle postpartum moves," Fit Pregnancy Magazine.

[392] "Why Exercise During Pregnancy?" womenshealth.gov.

[393] "Exercising While You're Pregnant," babyfit.com.

[394] Booth and Alpino.

[395] "Why Exercise During Pregnancy?" womenshealth.gov.

[396] Rich, "Organic fruits and vegetables work harder for their nutrients, *San Francisco Chronicle*, sfgate.com

[397] "Does It Pay to Buy Organic? For pregnant women and children, the benefits are worth the higher price," Business Week, businessweek.com.

[398] "Wise Use of Herbs and Vitamins During Pregnancy," childbirthsolutions.com.

[399] Ibid.

[400] "Vitamins and Minerals. What You Eat Is Just as Important as How Much You Eat," pregnancy-info.net.

[401] Roberts, 81–93.

[402] Ibid., 83.

[403] Mcdougall, 51.

[404] Roberts, 96.

[405] Interview with Dina Aronson, MS, RD.

[406] Mcdougall, 50.

[407] Challem, "Caution Urged with Vitamin A in Pregnancy—But Beta-Carotene Is Safe." The Nutrition Reporter Newsletter, thenutritionreporter.com.

[408] Roberts, 100–101.

[409] Interview with Dina Aronson, MS, RD.

[410] Ibid., 115–116.

[411] Ibid., 124–126.

[412] Cousens, 649.

[413] Davis and Vesanto, *Becoming Vegan*, 166.

[414] Cousens, 649.

[415] Roberts,123–124.

[416] Burch and Sachs, 57.

[417] Roberts, 117.

[418] Cousens, 649.

[419] Ibid., 647.

[420] Ibid., 642.

[421] Ibid., 642.

[422] Vincent, Beth, MHS, "The importance of DHA during pregnancy and breastfeeding," pregnancyandbaby.com.

[423] Cousens, 645.

[424] Interview with Dina Aronson, MS, RD.

[425] Delany, "Omega 3 Fat During Pregnancy," DrDelany.com.

[426] Raffelock, Roundtree, Hopkins and Block, *A Natural Guide to Pregnancy and Postpartum Health*, 132.

[427] Ibid., 135.

[428] Cousens, 650.

[429] Burch and Sachs, 55.

[430] Cousens, 635–639.

[431] "Breastfeeding Benefits from Top to Bottom," askdrsears.com.

[432] Huggins, "How breastfeeding benefits you and your baby," babycenter.com.

[433] "AAP Releases Revised Breastfeeding Recommendations," ap.org.

[434] Dermer and Montgomery, "Breastfeeding: Good for Babies, Mothers, and the Planet," medicalreporter.health.org.

[435] Burby, Leslie, "101 Reasons to Breastfeed Your Child," promom.org and Endocrine Regulations.

[436] Huggins, babycenter.com.

[437] Dermer and Montgomery, medicalreporter.health.org.

[438] Huggins, babycenter.com.

[439] Dermer and Montgomery, medicalreporter.health.org.

[440] Greene, "Benefits of Breastfeeding," drgreene.com.

[441] Dermer and Montgomery, medicalreporter.health.org.

[442] Huggins, "How breastfeeding benefits you and your baby," babycenter.com.

[443] "Benefits of Breastfeeding," United States Breastfeeding Committee, usbreastfeeding.org.

[444] Boyles, "Weight Gain Between Pregnancies Increases Risks," foxnews.com.

[445] "Benefits of Breastfeeding," usbreastfeeding.org.

[446] Burby, Promom.org Rosenblatt, "Prolonged lactation and endometrial cancer," *International Journal of Epidemiology*.

[447] Ibid., Heacock, "Influence of Breast vs. Formula Milk in Healthy Newborn Infants," *Journal of Pediatric Gastroenterology Nutrition*.

[448] Ibid., and Loesch, "Nutrition and dental decay in infants," *American Journal of Clinical Nutrition*.

[449] Ibid., Neiva, *Journal of Pediatrics*.

[450] Ibid., Piscane, "Breast-feeding and inguinal hernia," *Journal of Pediatrics*.

[451] Ibid., Freudenheim, "Exposure to breast milk in infancy and the risk of breast cancer," *International Journal of Epidemiology*

[452] "Benefits of Breastfeeding," usbreastfeeding.org.

[453] Burby, promom.org and Walker, *The Journal of Human Lactation*.

[454] "F.D.A Recalls of Baby Formula," breastfeeding.com.

[455] Osterweil, "Filthy Lucre." webmd.com.

[456] "Recalls and Field Corrections: Foods Class II," Enforcement report, fda.gov.

[457] Recalls and Field Corrections: Foods Class I," Enforcement report, fda.gov.

[458] "Bacteria Enterobacter Sakazakii," Reference.com.

[459] Defao, "Glass baby bottles making comeback. Stores selling out after health alarms raised about plastics," sfgate.com.

[460] "Baby Alert: Why Plastic Teethers & Bottles Are Bad," ecowise.com.

[461] Defao, "Glass baby bottles making comeback. Stores selling out after health alarms raised about plastics," sfgate.com.

[462] DeNoon, "Danger in Plastic Baby Bottles?" webmd.com.

[463] "Ask the fitness and nutrition experts," babyfit.com.

[464] Dermer and Montgomery, medicalreporter.health.org.

[465] Parpia Khan, "Maternal Nutrition during Breastfeeding," New Beginnings, lalecheleague.org.

[466] Dermer and Montgomery, medicalreporter.health.org.

[467] Burby, Promom.org and Kalwart, "Bone mineral loss during lactation," Journal of Obstetrics and Gynocology.

[468] Arcoverde, "World Breastfeeding Week. Breastfeeding: Nature's Way," waba.org.

[469] "Health news—alcohol lowers breast milk production," bupa.co.uk.

[470] Kirkpatrick, apparenting.com.

[471] Parpia, lalecheleague.org.

[472] Ibid.

[473] "Breast Milk Interactions Charts," babycenter.com.

[474] Zeretzke, "Allergies and the Breastfeeding Family," New Beginnings, lalecheleague.org.

[475] "Breast Milk Interactions Charts," babycenter.com.

[476] Dermer and Montgomery, medicalreporter.health.org.

[477] Parpia, Lalecheleague.org,

[478] Burby, promom.org and "Global Strategy for Infant and Young Child Feeding," World Health Organization in collaboration with UNICEF.

[479] "AAP Releases Revised Breastfeeding Recommendations," aap.org.

[480] Burby, promom.org.

[481] Burby, promom.org and Journal of the American Dietetic Association.

[482] Bernstein, "Soy Formula as Alternative to Breast Milk," life.familyeducation.com.

[483] "How Breast Milk Is Produced," babies.sutterhealth.org.

[484] DeFao, "Moms pay big for other mothers' milk. But doctors warn non-nursing women of health risk to babies." *San Francisco Chronicle*, sfgate.com.

[485] "Here's to Pickles and Ice Cream," medicinenet.com.

[486] Campbell and Campbell II, xv–368.

[487] "Cow's Milk Allergy versus Lactose Intolerance," nationaldairycouncil.org.

[488] "Vegetarian Diets for Children: Right from the Start," pcrm.org.

[489] "IFC Discusses a Study on Soy Infant Formula and Adult Health Outcomes," International Formula Council, Infantformula.org.

[490] Strom, Schinnar, Zeigler, Barnhart, Sammuel, Macones, Stallings, Drulis, Nelson, Hanson, "Exposure to Soy-Based Formula in Infancy and Endocrinological and Reproductive Outcomes in Young Adulthood," *Journal of the American Medical Association*, jama.org.

[491] Core, "Study Examines Long-Term Health Effects of Soy Infant Formula," *Agricultural Research Magazine*, ars.usda.gov.

[492] Kids Safe Chemical Act Empowers EPA to Require Chemical Testing," Environmental News Service, truthout.org.

[493] "Cancer-Causing Chemical Found in Children's Bath Products." Environmental Working Group, http://www.ewg.org/files/14-dioxane.pdf

[494] Ibid.

[495] Cik, "Five Problems with Baby Mattresses (toxic chemicals)," healthychild.com.

[496] Ibid.

[497] "What You Should Know About Chemicals in Your Cosmetics," Consumer Reports, safecosmetics.org.

[498] Waldman, "Ingredients in cosmetics, toys a safety concern," *The Wall Street Journal*, post-gazette.com.

[499] "What You Should Know About Chemicals in Your Cosmetics," safecosmetics.org.

[500] "Baby Care Products," The Learning and Developmental Disabilities Initiative, Iceh.org.

[501] "Johnson's Baby Lotion," Johnson & Johnson Consumer Companies, johnsonsbaby.com.

[502] Environmental Working Group's Skin Deep Cosmetic Safety Database," cosmeticdatabase.com.

[503] "Cosmetics and Anti-Aging Products—What's Safe During Pregnancy," womenshealthcaretopics.com.

[504] Bouchez, "Pregnancy Skin Care: Get That Glow," webmd.com.

[505] "Beauty Dos and Don'ts for Pregnant Women," ivillage.com.

[506] Dolan and Zissu, *The Complete Organic Pregnancy*, 242.

[507] "Diapers, Diapers & More Diapers. Cloth vs. Disposable," thenewparentsguide.com.

[508] Dolan and Zissu, 206.

[509] "Diapers, Diapers & More Diapers. Cloth vs. Disposable," thenewparentsguide.com.

[510] Matthiessen, "Mommy, Mama, Mutter: Motherhood Around the World." lifestyle.msn.com.

[511] Cik, Healthychild.com.

[512] "Hazardous Chemicals Found in a Wide Range of Baby Products," Environmental News Service, organicconsumers.org.

[513] Stallone and Jacobson, "Cheating Babies: Nutritional Quality and Cost of Commercial Baby Food," CSPI Reports, cspinet.org.

[514] "Stage by Stage, an Ingredient List for all Heinz Baby Food," heinzbaby.com.

[515] Stallone and Jacobson, "Cheating Babies: Nutritional Quality and Cost of Commercial Baby Food," CSPI Reports, cspinet.org.

[516] Telephone Interview to 1-800-4-GERBER

[517] Rodriguez and Greenfield, "Vaginal Bleeding After Delivery," drspock.com.

[518] "Postpartum Bleeding," epigee.org.

[519] Somer, 233.

[520] Oglesby,"Postpartum depression: More than 'baby blues,'" cnn.com.

[521] Somer, 233.

[522] "Postpartum Depression," med.umich.edu.

[523] "Postpartum Depression: Symptoms, Treatment, and Support," helpguide.org.

[524] Ibid.

[525] Ibid.

[526] Barnes, "Maternity Leave Helps Banish the Baby Blues," babyfit.com.

[527] Donovan, "Postpartum depression: Can nursing lessen its impact?" ivillage.com.

[528] "Baby Blues or Postpartum Depression," mommysmunchkins.com.

[529] "When do most couples start having sex again after their baby is born?" babycenter.com.

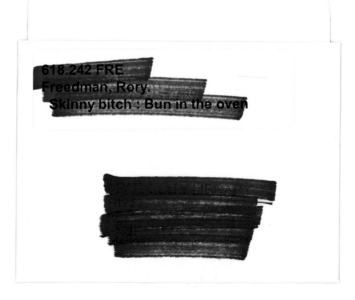